Register Now for Online Access to Your Book!

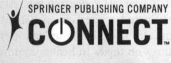

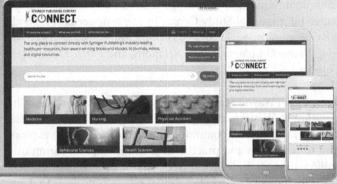

Videos and Podcasts included!

Your print purchase of *Communication and Care Coordination for the Palliative Care Team: A Handbook for Building and Maintaining Optimal Teams* **includes online access to the contents of your book—** increasing accessibility, portability, and searchability!

Access today at:

http://connect.springerpub.com/content/book/978-0-8261-5806-2 or scan the QR code at the right with your smartphone and enter the access code below.

Scan here for quick access.

RJHGF68H

SPRINGER PUBLISHING COMPANY

View all our products at springerpub.com

Rebecca S. Imes, PhD (University of Iowa), is associate professor of communication at Carroll University. With a lifelong interest in provider–patient relationships, she began her study of health communication at Tufts University School of Medicine and Emerson College, and she has been researching and teaching in this area for the past 20 years. Her research interests concern relationships in health contexts, and her work includes research on patient–family communication, provider–patient communication, and communication in high-functioning palliative care teams. She also lectures on topics in health communication in settings such as the Medical College of Wisconsin and the Bader International Study Center in Herstmonceux, England. She is published in *Health Communication*, *Journal of Health Communication*, *Journal of Family Communication*, *Psycho-Oncology*, *Family Relations*, and *Patient Education and Counseling*, among others.

Leah M. Omilion-Hodges, PhD (Wayne State University), is associate professor in the School of Communication at Western Michigan University. Her research fuses organizational communication with health communication, allowing her to explore questions that are relevant to academics and practitioners within applied communication contexts. Dr. Omilion-Hodges draws from her years of professional experience working in the healthcare industry to help her design research projects that are theoretically grounded but offer real-world insight for organizational members. Her primary areas of research include leader–member relationships, workgroup dynamics, and the employee experience within the palliative care setting. Her work has been published in *Leadership Quarterly*, *Management Communication Quarterly*, *Communication Yearbook: Annals of the International Communication Association*, *International Journal of Business Communication*, *Business and Professional Communication Quarterly*, and *Health Communication*, among others.

Jennifer D. B. Hester, DNP (The Christ Hospital Health Network), is a palliative care clinical nurse specialist practicing with a high-performing transdisciplinary team at The Christ Hospital in Cincinnati, Ohio. She earned a MS and DNP at the University of Colorado Health Sciences Center and is a board-certified APRN in both palliative care (ACHPN) and oncology (AOCNS). For the past 10 years, she has led the development and growth of a palliative care program that is recognized by The Joint Commission for Advanced Certification in Palliative Care. She serves as faculty for The Christ Hospital's Hospice and Palliative Medicine Fellowship Program. She has presented her work on the development of electronic health records for outcomes measurement in her field at the American Academy of Hospice and Palliative Medicine Annual Assemblies and the Center to Advance Palliative Care National Seminars. She is published in the *Clinical Journal of Oncology Nursing*.

COMMUNICATION AND CARE COORDINATION FOR THE PALLIATIVE CARE TEAM

A Handbook for Building and Maintaining Optimal Teams

Rebecca S. Imes, PhD

Leah M. Omilion-Hodges, PhD

Jennifer D. B. Hester, DNP

SPRINGER PUBLISHING COMPANY

Springer Publishing Company, LLC
11 West 42nd Street
New York, NY 10036
www.springerpub.com
http://connect.springerpub.com

Acquisitions Editor: Elizabeth Nieginski
Compositor: Amnet Systems

ISBN: 978-0-8261-5805-5
ebook ISBN: 978-0-8261-5806-2
Instructor's Case Studies ISBN: 978-0-8261-8921-9
Self-Care Plan Template ISBN: 978-0-8261-8917-2

DOI: 10.1891/9780826158062

Instructor's Materials: Qualified instructors may request supplements by emailing textbook@springerpub.com
A supplementary Self-Care Plan Template is available at springerpub.com/palliativecareteam

Visit https://connect.springerpub.com/content/book/978-0-8261-5806-2 to access accompanying videos and podcasts.

Printed by BnT

The author and the publisher of this Work have made every effort to use sources believed to be reliable to provide information that is accurate and compatible with the standards generally accepted at the time of publication. Because medical science is continually advancing, our knowledge base continues to expand. Therefore, as new information becomes available, changes in procedures become necessary. We recommend that the reader always consult current research and specific institutional policies before performing any clinical procedure. The author and publisher shall not be liable for any special, consequential, or exemplary damages resulting, in whole or in part, from the readers' use of, or reliance on, the information contained in this book. The publisher has no responsibility for the persistence or accuracy of URLs for external or third-party Internet websites referred to in this publication and does not guarantee that any content on such websites is, or will remain, accurate or appropriate.

Library of Congress Cataloging-in-Publication Data
Names: Imes, Rebecca S., author. | Omilion-Hodges, Leah M., author. |
  Hester, Jennifer D. B., author.
Title: Communication and care coordination for the palliative care team : a
  handbook for building and maintaining optimal teams / Rebecca S. Imes,
  Leah M. Omilion-Hodges, Jennifer D.B. Hester.
Description: New York, NY : Springer Publishing Company, LLC, [2021] |
  Includes bibliographical references and index.
Identifiers: LCCN 2019051660 (print) | LCCN 2019051661 (ebook) | ISBN
  9780826158055 (paperback) | ISBN 9780826158062 (ebook)
Subjects: MESH: Palliative Care | Patient Care Team | Communication |
  Interprofessional Relations | Patient-Centered Care
Classification: LCC R726.8 (print) | LCC R726.8 (ebook) | NLM WB 310 |
  DDC 616.02/9—dc23
LC record available at https://lccn.loc.gov/2019051660
LC ebook record available at https://lccn.loc.gov/2019051661

Rebecca S. Imes: https://orcid.org/0000-0002-8533-7272
Leah M. Omilion-Hodges: https://orcid.org/0000-0001-5574-5155
Jennifer D. B. Hester: https://orcid.org/0000-0002-9034-5963

Printed in the United States of America.

This book is dedicated to the legions of palliative care providers in all disciplines who perform such important, difficult work.

Additionally, Dr. Imes would like to thank the team at The Christ Hospital for allowing her access. She also appreciates her family's patience, love, and support and her daughter's help with organizing drafts.

Dr. Omilion-Hodges would like to thank her family and friends for their unyielding support, encouragement, and laughter. She would also like to thank the palliative care team at St. Joseph Mercy Oakland for opening her eyes to the significant and complex work of palliative care.

Dr. Hester is deeply grateful for her colleagues on the palliative care team for their willingness to approach the concept of teamwork with creativity and intention. She would like to thank Dr. Doug Smucker for his thoughtful partnership in building the team and Zoey Peterson for first introducing her to the concept of consensus work for creating intentional community. She also appreciates her husband's support and professional advice for this project.

CONTENTS

Foreword Andy E. Esch, MD, MBA   ix
Preface   xi
Acknowledgments   xv
Palliative Care Resources   xvi

1. Why We Need to Talk About Teams and
   Communication in Palliative Care   1

2. Who Are the Players? Exploring the Types of
   Palliative Care Providers   33

3. Formation and Maintenance of High-Performing
   Palliative Care Teams   61

4. Leading Palliative Care Teams   99

5. Interdisciplinary Palliative Care Team Meetings   133

6. Occupational Culture: Understanding the Role and
   Stigma of Palliative Care   161

7. Self-Care and Team Care in Emotional
   Labor–Intensive Positions   191

Index   229

FOREWORD

The U.S. health system was built to target and cure specific illnesses such as cancer or heart disease. However, in a health system in which technological advancement leads to departmental silos, we risk thinking of people as bundles of organs. A system that sets out to treat diseased organs and is not built to consider the person as a whole shortchanges the most important parts of the human experience to patients and families: quality of life and experience of care.

Treatment for people living with serious illness or multiple chronic conditions often involves so many physicians and other healthcare providers that it is impossible for one person to be aware of—let alone meet—the needs of patients and families. In this book, Dr. Imes and her colleagues reveal the answer to effective patient-centered care for serious illness, and that answer is palliative care. Palliative care is a team-based specialty focused on relieving the pain, symptoms, and suffering of patients living with serious illness and supporting their family members or caregivers. The focus is on the experience of living with disease and optimizing quality of life.

Palliative care uses a team of doctors, nurses, social workers, chaplains, and others working together to make patients and families aware that quality of life matters most and delivering on that promise. This book explores what it takes for palliative care teams to deliver high-quality patient-centered care that addresses all the complex real-world needs that patients and families experience. This is difficult work, and for teams to be effective, they need to be healthy and high functioning. Dr. Imes and her coauthors examine what goes into the formation, growth, and functioning of palliative care teams, touching on topics such as team makeup, team stressors, self-care of team members and cultivating resilience, and integration of palliative care teams in our complex, and in many ways broken, healthcare system.

The team-based nature of palliative care is perfectly designed for the future of healthcare and should serve as a model for the rest of the health system. There is no shortcut for addressing the gaps in care that too often result in patient suffering. Palliative care teams have decades of experience providing high-quality care that is focused on the person, not just the disease, and is delivered in a cost-effective, sustainable way. Palliative care lives in this intersection of cost sustainability and improved quality. This book helps us understand what it takes for palliative care teams to get there and stay there.

Andy E. Esch, MD, MBA
Consultant
Center to Advance Palliative Care
New York, New York

PREFACE

Palliative care continues to be a rapidly growing area of medicine. The fact that hospitals and health systems are devoting resources specifically geared toward the care of patients and families experiencing serious illness is an important and long-awaited turn for healthcare. Better yet, the awareness continues to grow, and research supports the idea that interdisciplinary palliative care teams are the optimal way to care for seriously ill patients. Yet, as Dr. David Weissman, founding editor of *The Journal of Palliative Care*, observes, this increasing demand for services may result in an integrated team devolving to a loosely connected group of health professionals. When this happens, the power of the team is lost. *Communication and Care Coordination for the Palliative Care Team* is designed to help you avoid common pitfalls while starting a team or correct issues in an already formed palliative care team. We want your team to do more than survive—we want you to thrive!

Unlike most books about palliative care, our text is geared toward equipping practicing healthcare professionals or healthcare students with practical solutions for working within complex, multifaceted palliative care teams. We base our text on the foundational idea that communication is at the heart of all relationships and interactions, and we use evidence-based analysis to connect ideas about forming and maintaining a high-performing palliative care team. Departing from the traditional foci of provider–patient rapport and pain and symptom management, we offer pragmatic solutions to common organizational headaches and unique palliative care team issues by helping practitioners consider the intricacies of interdisciplinary team dynamics, occupational culture, and self-care in emotional, labor-intensive positions. While this book will be especially attractive for the working palliative care professional, it will also be a useful socialization tool for medical and nursing schools, as well as graduate communication and social work programs and advanced undergraduate courses in health communication, nursing, and sociology.

The text's driving theme is an emphasis on the foundational nature of communication for individual and collective performance within palliative care teams. We frame communication as constitutive; in other words, our unique experience in our organization is based on how we approach communication in our interpersonal, group, and organizational relationships. Focus on the conscious use of communication to form and maintain productive work relationships is not a new concept. However, communication is most often framed as a tool to fix problems of accuracy in transmitting information, rather than as the underlying foundation upon which all relationships are based. Viewing communication as foundational encourages practitioners to switch perspectives from simply attempting to transmit a better message to being aware of the foundational nature of creating meaning between individuals. While transmission of a productive, effective message remains an important element of high-performing transdisciplinary teams, its power is lost when a well-constructed message goes awry. Evolving a transmission perspective to a foundational perspective makes communication more than a tool to be used in difficult situations and enables practitioners to be mindful of the communicative foundation upon which all their daily interactions are based. It is this mindfulness combined with the training to execute meaningful communication in teams that transforms teams from connected groups of health professionals to healthy, high-performing interdisciplinary and transdisciplinary teams.

The foundational view of communication is a particularly useful framework when merging a number of different specialties onto a single team. This is especially important in a working environment that has the additional stressors and pressures of helping patients and their loved ones to experience a good death. Arising from models for the delivery of holistic care, palliative care teams are composed of a wide variety of healthcare professionals who come together to fulfill the physical, psychosocial, emotional, logistical, and spiritual needs of patients and their loved ones. If these teams are strewn together haphazardly, there may be gaps in patient care, and more so, palliative care providers may find themselves victims of power struggles and may even be more susceptible to burnout. As palliative care clinicians already experience higher rates of burnout than other types of nonphysician clinicians (Kamal et al., 2017), team processes that exacerbate stress are likely to increase this high turnover rate. Even thoughtful team construction can lead to undesirable outcomes if team members do not understand the importance of proactive communication in team maintenance. Therefore, through the authors' shared professional and research expertise, we walk providers through team and leadership essentials based on principles of adept and mindful communication and through the ins and outs of cooperative team-based patient care, complete with concrete suggestions and activities for newly formed or existing teams to inspire even higher levels of patient care and provider satisfaction.

Communication and Care Coordination for the Palliative Care Team is designed to help you understand teams in the unique setting of palliative care. This text utilizes the following:

- Stories from nurses, social workers, physicians, patients, families, executives, chaplains, and pharmacists
- Pearls From the Field: Provider and team takeaways
- Best practices of team leaders
- Tips for individuals and palliative care teams to communicate with other providers, departments, and senior leadership
- Discussions on how to improve short-term and long-term team functioning
- Outlines to use as predictors of burnout for palliative care providers and teams
- Self-care and team-care suggestions
- A combination of recent research and theory in an accessible writing style

Also available are case study and self-care plan supplements, as well as videos of interviews with palliative care providers and palliative care team podcasts, in which a team discusses issues within the palliative care field. (Please see p. xvi for further details.)

Reference

Kamal, A., Bull, J., Swetz, K., Wolf, S., Shanafelt, T., & Myers, E. (2017). Future of the palliative care workforce: A preview to an impending crisis. *The American Journal of Medicine, 130*(2), 113–114.

An introductory podcast is available with online access of this title. Please see the instructions on the first page of the book for details on how to access and go to the preface.

ACKNOWLEDGMENTS

The authors are grateful to the following individuals for their assistance on this project. We appreciate Emily Gaggioli for her design of the graphics throughout this book, Morgan Clark for her help in proofreading, and Tierra Billings for her patience and assistance with the digital components. Rebecca appreciates the support of Carroll University, which provided her a sabbatical to collect data and further financial support to complete the book. She also appreciates the invaluable support of her colleagues through the writing process. Finally, Rebecca and Jennifer want to acknowledge and thank their friends and faculty from their Nebraska Wesleyan University days as well as their family, friends, and teachers from their hometown of Gering, Nebraska. As we always say, we grew up with the best people. Without those foundational relationships forged long ago in our small town, this book would not have been possible.

PALLIATIVE CARE RESOURCES

Communication and Care Coordinator for the Palliative Care Team includes a robust resources package.

Each chapter of this text includes a supplementary podcast. These resources may be accessed via connect.springerpub.com/content/book/978-0-8261-5806-2.

Supplementary videos are also available:

- *Palliative Care: It Takes a Team*, presenting a physician's perspective from Dr. Doug Smucker. (This video may be accessed at connect.springerpub. com/content/book/978-0-8261-5806-2/ch01.)
- *Right Care at the Right Time*, presenting a social worker's perspective from Marjorie Rentz. (This video may be accessed at connect.springerpub.com/ content/book/978-0-8261-5806-2/ch02.)
- *Everybody Overlaps in an Interdisciplinary Team*, presenting a physician's perspective from Dr. Elizabeth Grady. This video may be accessed at connect.springerpub.com/content/book/978-0-8261-5806-2/ch03.)

A Self-Care Plan Template may be accessed via connect.springerpub.com/ content/book/978-0-8261-5806-2/ch07. (This resource may also be accessed at Springerpub.com/palliativecareteam.)

Qualified instructors may obtain access to a supplemental Case Study by emailing textbook@springerpub.com.

CHAPTER 1

WHY WE NEED TO TALK ABOUT TEAMS AND COMMUNICATION IN PALLIATIVE CARE

Introduction

Palliative care is one of the fastest growing areas of medicine. This vital field focuses on the care of seriously ill patients and their families. Team-based care has proven to be very effective in palliative care, and hospitals and health systems are turning toward this practice in ever greater numbers. However, many palliative care providers—physicians, APRNs, registered nurses, social workers, chaplains, and pharmacists—have limited experience working on a sustained, daily basis with colleagues outside of their discipline. When a team struggles to work together well, that stress compounds the already stressful environment that surrounds the care of the seriously ill. That compounded stress can lead to team turnover as members leave for other areas of practice or leave the field altogether. Given the importance of palliative care to families and to healthcare systems and hospitals, it is imperative that we find a way to help teams survive and thrive. Although often overlooked, a focus on interpersonal, team, and organizational communication can set a solid foundation on which teams can do just that—thrive as a team while doing the important work of caring for patients and families.

Negative Palliative Care Experience

Physician Experience: On a weekly basis, I'll have other physicians cut in line in the doctor's dining room and make remarks like "It's not like you need to rush to save anyone" or "It must be nice not to have to deal with an OR schedule." There's one guy in particular, a cardiologist, who will not only cut in front of me and then intentionally take as much time as is humanly possible to make a salad, but he'll also take

A podcast to accompany this chapter is available with online access of this title. Please see the instructions on the first page of the book for details on how to access and go to Chapter 1.

the newspaper right out of my hands and say "It's amazing you don't have this on 6 [location of the palliative care unit]. I don't know what you do with all of that time when you're babysitting the dying."

Positive Palliative Care Experience

Physician Experience: *This is the best team I've ever worked on. I mean, they're phenomenal. I think the other thing that really makes this work in a very positive way [is something] that maybe some other teams [at the hospital] have trouble connecting is that this is really meaningful work. And sometimes you may lose sight of the impact that has on team satisfaction; then you see one of your colleagues really do some amazing things with the family, and you see the outcome of that. You realize that you made a difference. You get to feel that and experience that. Every time I'm on this [palliative care team] service that happens. I can't say that happens on every team I'm on. Those are things that offset the draining portion of it [palliative care]. It's recognizing "This was heading down a path that could have been really bad, and we made a difference." It's very emotionally engaging, and you feel drained sometimes, but there is also this filling of the well again by your colleagues as well as just the meaning of the work.*

The Growth Trajectory of Palliative Care

The Center to Advance Palliative Care (CAPC) estimates that 12 million adults and 400,000 children in the United States are living with a serious disease, and that number is expected to double in the next 25 years (CAPC, 2018). Palliative care is specialized medical care for people with serious illnesses that is focused on the relief of symptoms, pain, and stress of a serious illness—whatever the stage of disease. In a best-practice scenario, this type of care is provided by an interdisciplinary team, usually comprised of physicians, nurses, social workers, and chaplains (CAPC, 2019b). Unlike hospice, which is end-of-life care for terminally ill patients, palliative care requires no enrollment or benefit choice and can be provided concurrently with curative treatment (National Consensus Project Clinical Practice Guidelines for Quality Palliative Care [NCP Guidelines], 2018; World Health Organization [WHO], 2017). The development of hospital-based palliative care services has been one of the most rapidly growing trends in the past 15 years as, in addition to the improvement of patient and family care, good palliative care teams (PCTs) provide cost savings to their hospitals (McCarthy, Robinson, Huq, Philastre, & Fine, 2015). CAPC, founded in 1999, continues to see growth in membership and conference participation (Meier, 2019 podcast). Thus, even though "payment cuts for the chronically ill and elderly are increasing" (Candrian, 2015, p. 732), palliative care development and utilization in hospitals is likely to continue its current trajectory.

Why Focus on Teams and Communication in Palliative Care?

In *Clinical Practice Guidelines for Quality Palliative Care*, Fourth Edition (NCP, 2018), the first section of the best-practice guidelines is devoted to the necessity of quality interdisciplinary teams. The list is comprehensive and mentions team communication numerous times. While it is not uncommon to see "good communication" listed as an important component of great healthcare, it is uncommon for that standard to be followed with research and ideas on how to recognize, teach, and perform good interpersonal, team, and organizational communication in healthcare settings. This book is the resource to help organizations form and/or maintain high-performing PCTs that can meet these guidelines. Combining the research on palliative care, high-performing teams, and healthcare organizational culture, this book uses original data sets, peer-reviewed literature, and national data banks to help you form a PCT or to transform your current team into one with less turnover. This book can help you to mindfully create a new PCT or enhance an already formed PCT in a way that relies on teamwork to help team members thrive in the sometimes difficult world of palliative care.

While teams are a newer way of organizing in many areas of healthcare, they are becoming the standard for palliative care. PCTs model holistic care through assembling multiple disciplines to work together to care for patients and families. Teams are important in palliative care, as teams gather the necessary resources of the disciplines of physicians, nurses, social workers, chaplains, and pharmacists to offer the best possible patient care. In addition, a well-functioning team has the added benefit of making better decisions and avoiding member burnout.

It is likely that you work in palliative care because you believe that providing excellent palliative care is essential to the well-being of patients, families, and healthcare systems. In health systems where the focus has long been on curing and ideas of a *good death* have often been framed as "giving up," palliative care providers fulfill the ethical and moral obligation to care for patients and families experiencing serious illness regardless of the possibility of curing that illness. Given the swift rise of palliative care in hospital systems, this book considers three truths in palliative care:

1. The demand for palliative care continues to grow.
2. The challenge of delivering excellent palliative care is best met through interdisciplinary teams.
3. Teams function best when they make intentional communication a priority.

Palliative Care Truth No. 1: Increasing Demand for Palliative Care

As palliative care continues its meteoric rise, devoting time, energy, and money to developing high-performing PCTs is a worthwhile investment. The palliative care subspecialty holds a unique role in the illness trajectory in that it focuses entirely on the relief of suffering and improvement of quality of life within the context of a serious illness. Recognition that palliative care results in improved quality of care and reduced cost has led to health systems' investment in the development of palliative care programs. Access to palliative care for seriously ill patients and their families is increasingly recognized as a clinical and moral imperative (Institute of Medicine [IOM], 2014). With professional guidelines such as those by the American Society of Clinical Oncology (ASCO) and disease-specific accreditation programs requiring early and routine concurrent palliative care, it has become increasingly clear that the need for palliative care will continue to outpace access to specialty palliative care clinicians (Compton-Phillips & Mohta, 2019; Quill & Abernathy, 2013).

As healthcare systems work to meet the complex needs of seriously ill patients with the recognition of an impending workforce shortage of specialty-trained palliative care providers (Kamal et al., 2017), there is an increasingly urgent call to promote primary palliative care, which is delivered by healthcare professionals—not palliative care specialists—such as primary care and disease-oriented clinicians (e.g., oncologists and cardiologists) as well as nurses, social workers, pharmacists, chaplains, and others who care for seriously ill patients and their families but are not specialty trained in palliative care (IOM, 2014).

According to Quill and Abernathy (2013), primary palliative care includes basic competency in:

- Pain and symptom management
- Depression and anxiety management
- Communication about prognosis, goals of treatment, suffering, and advance care planning

Specialty palliative care, provided by skilled and highly trained professionals, is required for the management of:

- Refractory pain and symptoms
- Complex depression, anxiety, grief, and existential distress
- Conflict resolution within families, between families and the treating teams, and among treatment teams
- Assistance with cases of medical futility

While the roles between providers of primary- and specialty-level palliative care will inevitably blur at times, the need for highly trained, dedicated PCTs to address the complex care needs of seriously ill patients and their families will remain paramount. In addition to providing direct care, specialty-level palliative care providers are also called upon to transform serious illness care through mentorship and training of all care providers on basic pain and symptom management and communication skills (i.e., CAPC Tipping Point Challenge, 2019). This quickly growing area of clinical care is here to stay. Given that a 2019 report on the results of the Catalyst Insights Council survey found that while "the great majority of organizations have a palliative or end-of-life care program, 60% of patients who would benefit from such services don't receive them" (Compton-Phillips & Mohta, 2019), the rate of growth in palliative care has not yet met the need. Additionally, the demand for palliative care will only continue to grow due to aging populations and improved clinical outcomes for seriously ill patients.

Aging Population

In 2030, the last of the baby boomers will turn 65. The U.S. Census Bureau predicts that by 2035, the number of people over 65 will outnumber the number of children under 18 for the first time in the history of the United States. As those over 65 use health services at much higher rates (e.g., May et al., 2018) than the rest of the population, the demand for palliative care professionals will rise. The public will demand the services and hospitals will look to PCTs to help keep expenditures under control. Approximately half of palliative care use is from patients between the ages of 65 and 85 (National Palliative Care Registry, 2017). Many members of this aging population have one or more chronic diseases. According to the Centers for Disease Control and Prevention (CDC, 2019), 60% of adults in the United States have one chronic disease, and 42% of U.S. adults have two or more. The leading chronic diseases in U.S. adults include the following:

- Heart disease
- Cancer
- Chronic lung disease
- Stroke
- Alzheimer's disease
- Diabetes
- Chronic kidney disease

These diseases are the leading causes of death and disability in the United States and are the primary drivers of the nation's $3.3 billion in annual healthcare costs. Among those aged 65 to 85, the population with the highest use of palliative care, two thirds of patients have multiple chronic conditions. So what does this mean for palliative care? It means that the medical specialty is likely to continue growing at exponential rates, and that, in turn, means that individual providers, teams, and organizations need to be equipped to offer patient-centered care in the face of the increased demand.

Improved Clinical Outcomes

The growing use of palliative care in the United States points to a sizable shift in Western medicine—an understanding that the quality of a patient's life is at least as important as the number of years a patient lives. Considerable evidence (Box 1.1) exists showing that palliative care improves clinical outcomes throughout the trajectory of serious illness care.

BOX 1.1

EVIDENCE FOR IMPROVED OUTCOMES WITH PALLIATIVE CARE

Davis et al. (2015)

A meta-analysis of outpatient and home palliative care studies found that despite some methodological concerns, the current state of palliative care research supports the conclusion that early outpatient and home palliative care may improve the patient's quality of life.

Fitzpatrick et al. (2018)

"Early intervention with inpatient palliative care consultation (within 3 days) correlated with financial benefit as well as earlier referral to more appropriate levels of care" (CAPC-Research in the field, 2019a).

Kerr et al. (2014)

Among patients with life-limiting or serious illness enrolled in a blended outpatient/home palliative care program, symptomology improved in six domains: anxiety, appetite, dyspnea, well-being, depression, and nausea.

Kavalieratos et al. (2016)

A meta-analysis found that palliative care was associated with statistically and clinically significant improvements in both patient quality of life (QOL) and symptom burden at the 1- to 3-month follow-up. Additionally, palliative care was associated consistently with improvements in advance care planning, patient and caregiver satisfaction, and lower healthcare utilization.

See the Center to Advance Palliative Care's (CAPC) website on Research in the Field (https://registry.capc.org/metrics-resources/research-in-the-field) for more article suggestions to help make your case for starting, growing, and maintaining palliative care teams in your organization.

BOX 1.2

A PHYSICIAN REFLECTS: PALLIATIVE CARE IS DESERVING OF HOSPITAL RESOURCES

A colleague from neurology approached me in a highly agitated state after he found out that my palliative group received permission for new hires and promotional materials. He could not come to grips with this. He could not rationalize why the organization would give money to a program that was not revenue generating. The problem with this is that making money is prized over ethical obligation. I didn't become a doctor to make an organization rich. I went into palliative care because caring for people is the right thing to do (Omilion-Hodges & Swords, 2017).

A recent nuance of that shift is that the quality of a patient's death is also important (Box 1.2). Evidence of this shift includes the creation of numerous assessment measures, which were systematically studied by Hales, Zimmerman, and Rubin (2010). They found the Quality of Death and Dying Scale (QODD) to be the most used and best validated. One consideration for this measure is that it is used retrospectively for the family to consider the last days of the loved one's life. In other words, when families are in the midst of dealing with serious illness, they do not necessarily make the decisions that they will later wish they had made. Physician and author Atul Gawande reflects on this with the spouse of a former patient in the PBS *Frontline* episode, Being Mortal (Jennings, 2015). As Boston surgeon Dr. Gawande notes, due to the patient and family focus on treatment, he held back from encouraging them to focus on the time the patient had remaining. The patient's husband now also speaks of their hyperfocus on treatment and how he wishes they would have chosen a palliative path earlier and enjoyed more of her ending days together.

Growth of PCTs

Given the evidence of need for specialized seriously ill care and the possibilities of significant fiscal savings for hospitals and health systems, the number of PCTs is increasing in clinical practice. J. Andrew Billings issued a call to arms in 2002, stating, "Our focus for the moment should be in developing skilled interdisciplinary teams that provide high-quality, coordinated care across settings" (p. 298). Many healthcare systems are working to answer that call. Nearly 90% of hospitals with 300 or more beds (Dumanovsky et al., 2016) and 79% of hospitals with 50 or more beds (CAPC, 2018) have specialty palliative care programs. At least 1,852 sites of service in the United States offer specialized palliative care (CAPC, 2018). While this is encouraging, very few of these hospitals have sufficient staffing for their programs (Spetz et al., 2016). Ledford, Canzona, Cafferty, and Kalish (2016) also point out that the majority of palliative care is offered by internists without specific palliative care training or the support of a PCT. So while programs are growing, the training of experts in palliative care is not keeping pace. The 2014 IOM report, *Dying in America*, found "inadequate numbers of palliative care specialists and too little palliative care knowledge among other clinicians who care for individuals with serious advanced illness" (p. 2). With just 3% of U.S. hospitals holding certification in specialized palliative care (CAPC, 2018), the growth and training opportunities for PCTs are numerous.

▶ Palliative Care Truth No. 2: The Challenge of Providing Excellent Palliative Care is Best Met through Interdisciplinary Teams

The team model harnesses the expertise of multiple disciplines into a single care team. These teams benefit from the perspectives of the different disciplines and, if they manage to form a high-performing team, can develop a model of learning and shared care among team members that benefits both the team and the patients and families with whom the team works. Some teams form a minimally competent model, and while they work together, they do not work together particularly well. Table 1.1 delineates the minimally performing team from the high-performing team. This chart illustrates how an idea that sounds simple is often very difficult to construct—how do you form a great team? This book will assist you with the answer to that question.

Fiscal Savings for Hospitals

While it is better for care providers to have a high-performing team, why should hospitals and healthcare systems be motivated to invest in helping to create high-performing teams rather than remaining satisfied with minimally performing teams? If palliative care models were not financially beneficial for hospitals, it

---

▶ An accompanying video, Palliative Care: It Takes a Team, presenting a physician's perspective from Dr. Doug Smucker, may be accessed at connect.springerpub.com/content/book/978-0-8261-5806-2/ch01.

TABLE 1.1 Minimally Versus High-Performing Palliative Care Teams (PCTs)

HIGH-PERFORMING PCTs	MINIMALLY PERFORMING PCTs
Proactive process to identity patients appropriate for PCT referrals	Reactive patient identification process for PCT involvement
Flexible approaches to pain management	Standardized approach to pain management
Clear roles and responsibilities of team members	Confusing roles and unclear responsibilities for team members
High patient and family engagement possible early in the disease process	Burdensome time and resource pressures due to late and limited engagement with family and patient
Good understanding of PCT in the context of the hospital organization	Limited understanding of how the PCT fits in the hospital context
Great teamwork between experts	Experts who work together

SOURCE: Adapted from Hackett, J., Ziegler, L., Godfrey, M., Foy, R., & Bennett, M. I. (2018). Primary palliative care team perspectives on coordinating and managing people with advanced cancer in the community: A qualitative study. *BMC Family Practice, 19*, 177. doi:10.1186/s12875-018-0861-z; Imes, R. S., & Hester, J. (2015). *Unintended intentional community at work: Applying a new lens to guide the formation and maintenance of transdisciplinary teams.* Paper presented at the National Communication Association Annual Convention, Las Vegas; Omilion-Hodges, L. M., & Baker, C. R. (2017). Communicating leader-member relationship quality: The development of leader communication exchange scales to measure relationship building and maintenance through the exchange of communication-based goods. *International Journal of Business Communication, 54*(2), 115–145. doi:10.1177/2329488416687052

is unlikely that the model would have survived, yet the number of hospitals with palliative care and patients utilizing palliative care services continues to surge. Palliative care can be a difficult concept for some medical specialties to understand because PCTs do not *make* money for the hospital; PCTs *save* money for the hospital (Box 1.3). These fiscal savings are another kind of value work provided by palliative care—the human value of caring for seriously ill people and economic value of saving hospitals' money through lower use of EDs and ICUs for palliative patients. While the humanity element is often cited by palliative care advocates as the primary argument for supporting PCTs in hospitals, fiscal savings for hospitals and systems make another compelling argument for building and supporting PCTs (Box 1.4). In fact, one source predicts that increased use of palliative care will save the U.S. healthcare system over $103 billion before 2040 (Parker, 2019).

Mounting evidence shows that interdisciplinary PCTs save hospitals more money than those that have palliative care through a single discipline. For

BOX 1.3

STUDIES SHOW FISCAL SAVINGS FOR HOSPITALS WITH PALLIATIVE CARE

May et al. (2017)

This study found that palliative care does save money over usual care.

- Three primary drivers of savings are lower room and board costs and fewer imaging and laboratory tests. In the United States, 63% of the savings came from lower room and board and 37% from "reduced intensity of service" (p. 382).

- Pharmacy costs (the other high driver of costs in hospitals) were unchanged between usual care and palliative-involved care.

- Early palliative care involvement is a good predictor of savings. This study found a predictable correlation between late palliative care involvement and higher length of stay (LOS) and intensity of service costs.

Meier et al. (2017)

Palliative care in general can reduce healthcare costs by more than $4,000 per patient. It can also reduce the frequency of 911 calls, ED visits, and unnecessary hospitalizations.

May et al. (2018)

In the specific case of oncology there was a reduction in cost of care with early palliative care involvement for diagnoses of primary cancer with comorbidities. Of those cases, the greatest reduction was found when a palliative care consultation occurred within three days of hospital admission for patients with a primary cancer and four or more comorbidities (p. 827).

Smith et al. (2012)

Kaiser Permanente, an insurer and provider of medical care for over 12 million members (https://share.kaiserpermanente.org/about-us/about-kaiser-permanente), designed palliative care standards in all areas for which Kaiser Permanente has a significant market share. The adoption was based on a randomized controlled trial that demonstrated savings of $5,000 to $7,000 per person.

example, a study of two similar Ohio hospitals within the same health system found that a PCT with physicians and APRNs resulted in earlier referrals and shorter lengths of stay, which resulted in greater cost savings for the hospital than the APRN-only team (Kousaie & von Gunten, 2017, p. 1313). The authors attribute the difference in lengths of stay to the difference in communication between

BOX 1.4

A PHYSICIAN REFLECTS: RETURN ON INVESTMENT
Our APRN has done a wonderful job putting the data together showing the administration what exactly they've put their money into, and now the administration understands. They truly bought into our plan, and when we ask for more, they can see the data. It's not just because we think we need it—we can prove to them the return on investment.

nurses and physicians depending on whether they were part of the same team. When they were not, the communication was characterized as indirect, and the authors discovered that the nurses were less likely to challenge the physician concerning the plan of care. When nurses and physicians were on the same PCT, the communication appeared more direct with all parties contributing to the conversation and adapting the plan. The authors identify this more direct, engaged team communication as the reason for the shortened post-consult lengths of stay, which was half that of the nurse-only team.

In addition to better team discussions, a fully staffed team can help avoid one of the pitfalls of palliative care—burnout. For example, a fully staffed team can make time for team members to do some of what helps them thrive in palliative care. In an underresourced team, the problem is compounded when staff burns out from, for example, only doing discharge planning. Now the team is down a person and trying to hire. If the team changes nothing, they know that the situation is likely to come up again. While changes in staffing models requiring new ways to think about billing may be difficult conversations to begin for health organizations, the data support interdisciplinary models. A good prediction tool can help the argument for a PCT. The CAPC provides a financial calculator on their website (https://www.capc.org/impact-calculator). See an example of one hospital's use of the impact calculator (Exhibit 1.1). This tool can assist teams in making hiring arguments to their administrators.

Scharf, Geist Martin, Cosgriff-Hernandez, and Moore (2012) study integrative medicine, which is another area of medicine that requires an expanded way of thinking about personnel organizing and billing. They remind us that "trailblazing integrative medicine includes a multitude of challenges that require novel ways of thinking" (p. 438). As the data show, teams are an excellent way to care for seriously ill patients while saving hospitals money. This indicates that the work that is necessary to create new structures is worth the effort.

EXHIBIT 1.1

CENTER TO ADVANCE PALLIATIVE CARE IMPACT CALCULATOR

Estimated Financial Impact: An Example of Direct Cost Savings Based on One Hospital's Data

DESCRIPTION	EXAMPLE*
Estimated Average Cost per FTE Including Benefits With IDT Mix	$160,000
Estimated Team Costs (Staffing FTE x Average Cost)	$1,184,000
Estimated Billing Revenue (Part B Professional at CMS 2017 Rates	$509,290
Net Investment or Subsidy Needed (Staffing Costs- Billing Revenue)	$674,710
Estimated Direct Cost Savings per Case (Episode of Care)	$3,274
Expected Cost Savings Before Deducting Net Investment	$4,953,562
Expected Annual Direct Cost Savings (Savings - Investments)	$4,278,852

*Example data drawn from a large teaching hospital.

CMS, Centers for Medicare & Medicaid Services; FTE, full-time equivalent; IDT, interdisciplinary team.

SOURCE: Center to Advance Palliative Care. *CAPC impact calculator.* Retrieved from https://www.capc.org/impact-calculator/

Palliative Care Truth No. 3: Teams Function Best When They Make Intentional Communication a Priority

Palliative care is really hard work. Working with seriously ill patients and families with complex problems in a complex system can be draining. PCT colleagues Atayee and Edmonds (2018) remind us that labeling something as hard work is often frowned upon in the medical and pharmacy fields because "then it means we are complaining and don't care about our patients ... but the fact is that doing good palliative care is hard ... more than this, working as a team is hard" (p. 1386). Difficulties in providing palliative care on PCTs include the following:

■   Caring for patients with serious illness
■   Assisting families of patients with serious illness

- Dealing with grief as a provider
- Working in a culture of healthcare that may stigmatize palliative care as "giving up"
- Relating to team members with different personalities, from different disciplines, and with different underlying assumptions of how groups work together
- Embedding teams in hospital environments that have long worked under organizational structures of separation rather than interdisciplinary models

Given all these challenges, it may seem easier to forget about the team aspects and simply focus on patient care. However, the data show that interdisciplinary models are the best way to provide efficacious palliative care. Thus, focusing on the team must be a priority, and focusing on the team means focusing on communication. Watson, Heatley, Gallois, and Kruske (2016) found that "communication is perceived to be pivotal to collaborative practice. Nonetheless, the abilities and perceptions of care providers about communication can create difficulty in the application of collaborative practice" (p. 405). Klarare et al. elaborate on the importance of collaboration for the self-worth of individual collaborators, saying "that is crucial. No one wants to feel that 'I am replaceable' and that nothing changes even if I disappear.... You need to feel that it is good that you are here, because you bring us closer to our goal" (2013, p. 1066). With a strong focus on intentional communication for team building and maintenance, the hard work of caring for seriously ill patients and their families is less likely to be compounded by collaborative communication issues. When teams make communication a priority, even times of conflict are resolved faster and have few, if any, negative outcomes for the team environment.

To build PCTs that survive and thrive, a deep understanding of team and organizational communication is required. In fact, professional communication skills for healthcare providers is a topic that gets more attention with each passing year. In 2013, the Health Professionals Core Communication Curriculum (HPCCC) published their consensus learning objectives for medical education in Europe (Bachmann et al., 2013). In addition to an extensive section on provider–patient communication, the report includes a section devoted to communication on healthcare teams with subsections of teamwork and professional communication, leadership, and professional communication and management.

In the United States, similar communication deficits are noted. Nussbaum and Fisher (2009) define communicatively competent people as "individuals whose skills enable him or her to adapt to the challenges of the situation and, thus, have a better chance of completing a productive and satisfying interaction" (p. 199). Unfortunately, advanced communication skills were the most reported skill lacking among the people hired by community-based palliative care leaders (Dudley, Chapman, & Spetz, 2018). A 2018 study by Fulmer et al. found that only 29% of physicians reported formal training in how to conduct end-of-life conversations and 46% of the sample reported feelings of uncertainty about what to say in such conversations. Without adept communication, it becomes more challenging for providers to manage the emotional labor associated with the profession in addition to successfully navigating team conflict, status struggles, or successfully arguing for additional organizational resources. To better navigate these tensions, a good understanding of the foundational role of communication in relationships and workplace environments is necessary.

Foundational Role of Communication

Communication is often acknowledged as vital for teams and interpersonal interactions and yet is also often described in simplistic terms of how information is transmitted. Given all of the struggles that involve communication, it is useful to think of the foundational nature of communication as meaning making. A lingering misconception about communication is that it is simply a tool to pull out when someone would like to (a) get his or her way or (b) use it to clarify misunderstandings. This is a very simplistic view of communication. Focusing on communication as transmission can clear up misunderstandings if someone simply did not hear the other person correctly. In those situations, repeating or choosing a different channel of communication (i.e., avoiding texting when emotional nuance is a part of the message) can clear up the misunderstanding. However, when organizations cite "communication problems," the issue is usually one of meaning making between two or more people. In those situations, the preceding solutions do not work. If there is a value disagreement at the heart of a conflict, simply restating it louder and more slowly will not solve the conflict. For example:

- "I don't want to hire more people in palliative because palliative is about quitting. It's about giving up, and I don't want our patients to think we would give up on them! So we should use the funds to hire another APRN for my department because we are involved in actually curing patients."
- "'Just' a nurse?! Did you hear him say that I'm 'just' a nurse? I'm the one who caught three big medical mistakes last year!"

A more sophisticated view is to consider communication as a foundation. Without a solid foundation, homes sustain structural damage and cannot provide shelter. Without a solid foundation, marriages and relationships tend to crumble under everyday pressures and stressors. Neither of the preceding examples is simply a situation of not hearing someone correctly. Both show a difference in value and a difference in cultural communication expectation. Restating the same claim will not resolve these differences—both parties need to collaboratively communicate to try and get on the same page. Even with great communication, they may not agree, but they will better understand the other person's point of view.

Viewing communication as foundational suggests that it becomes the predominate lens for navigating and facilitating relationships, delivery of patient care, and traversing organizational life.

What the Foundational Role of Communication Looks Like in the Healthcare Environment

- **Intentional language usage:** Often, we are not fully aware of how our word choices may impact others. One of the authors worked on a healthcare team where her manager would refer to the team as "just my staff" and the administrative assistant as "just a secretary." The manager would most commonly do this when she was interacting with peers at her level or with organizational members at higher levels. Yet, when the manager communicated with the team without any higher status members present, she would call them her "dream team" and her "rock stars." No one, at any level, would ever like to be referred to as *just* a _____ (nurse/social worker/chaplain/physician).

  Additionally, the use of pejorative terms, such as *staff* instead of *team* and *secretary* instead of the more commonly used *administrative assistant*, can also put undue stress on individuals and negatively impact team lead–member relationships and team dynamics. The moral of the story is that language is powerful and can be used inclusively to fortify relationships or can inadvertently (or worse yet, intentionally) be used to stress status and power distinctions. The latter has resulted in a long history of medical errors and mishaps because exclusive language that stresses power differences and hierarchies can result in reduced interaction or the absence of communication (Lingard, Whyte, & Regehr, 2009; Makary & Daniel, 2016; Sutcliffe, Lewton, & Rosenthal, 2004).

- **Active listening:** The concept of active listening is quite simple—being present and engaged while listening to another. This may be in a hallway conversation with a peer, in a team meeting, or when engaging with a patient. Though it is easy to grasp theoretically, active listening requires practice, discipline, and trust. It may be easy to see how learning to remain in the present moment can take discipline and practice as we learn how to quiet our own thoughts as we fully consider the setting or context, the other individual's needs or goals, and our role in the situation (Omilion-Hodges & Swords, 2017). However, the role of trust may not be as obvious. When we engage in active listening in order to be present and to suspend our own desires and goals, we need to trust that others will return the favor. This is especially challenging in moments of conflict, if we are angry, fearful, or upset. In these moments, it is much easier to appear as though we are listening and instead silently work on our own rebuttal. Yet, doing so does not allow us to hear the other's perspective or point of view and, therefore, may result in a missed opportunity for understanding.

Active listening also includes asking questions, paraphrasing, and demonstrating affirming body language. Asking questions indicates that we have been attentive, whereas paraphrasing allows us to verify that we have interpreted or understood the other's perspective. Affirming body language includes making eye contact, facing the other person with open posture (uncrossing arms, leaning in to the speaker, and ignoring distractions), and nodding. This can be especially challenging in the fast-paced healthcare environment where phones, alarms, and hallway chatter create consistent background noise.

■ **Other-oriented approach:** This foundational communication tactic means a sincere attempt to understand before trying to be understood. An other-oriented approach also involves empathy in addition to intentional language usage and active listening. Especially in situations that involve disagreements or are riddled with pressure (a patient crashing), it can feel as though the only way to address or resolve the situation is by shouting our needs or demands until they are met. We can feel like no one is listening and necessary steps are being missed.

An other-oriented approach also means taking a step back to consider the bigger picture in terms of everyone's needs and goals. After doing so, it becomes easier to communicate effectively to make a plan that addresses the most pressing concerns first, while being mindful of secondary and tertiary steps. Even one person on a team who successfully enacts the other-oriented approach can help to calm the situation and help members reorient to focus on the conversation, task, or challenge at hand.

■ **Meaning-centered approach:** Adopting a meaning-centered approach to communication involves mastering intentional language, active listening, and an other-oriented approach. A meaning-centered view is the most complex and the most impactful as it requires individuals to be accountable for the ways in which they communicate. This includes being responsible for sensitive language choices, verifying that they are interpreting others' messages as they are intended, and demonstrating patience and skill in navigating complex or challenging situations by hearing and addressing others' concerns before privileging their own.

Additionally, a meaning-centered approach can include attempting to hear what someone means rather than what they are saying and considering how a person may change their communication tendencies depending on the situation. For example, while a team member may be saying they agree with the prevailing opinion, but their arms are crossed and they are fidgeting in their seat, an individual enacting a meaning-centered approach to communication may say "While it sounds like we're in general agreement, is there another possible option or consequence that we have not yet considered?" This aligns with suggestions forwarded in Chapter 5, Interdisciplinary Palliative Care Team Meetings. In sum, a meaning-centered approach encourages team members to consider the following while collaborating to deliver patient-centered care:

-Members' unique roles

-Situational goals

-Time and resource constraints

-Using intentional communication to play to individual strengths

-Using intentional communication to fortify team relationships

In summary, viewing communication as foundational empowers providers to be responsible for not only *what* they communicate but also *how* they communicate in the workplace. This is even more important in interdisciplinary and transdisciplinary teams where varied occupational training experiences often lead clinicians to use different language, make different assumptions, and employ different approaches to problem-solving. Yet, by modeling foundational communication skills, providers are equipped to successfully navigate these differences while maintaining a focus on patient-centered care and their own goals and specific responsibilities. One palliative care physician found that in the five years since his PCT was established, some positive changes in communication and structural changes in paperwork are directly related to the work of his team:

I work with internal medicine residents and they have patterned their communication style with families after what we do on this team. And the family medicine residents truly see us as a part of their team now. I was just reviewing a bunch of order sets for oncology and noticed they redid their chemo order sets and now there is checkmark for a palliative care consult—so it is no longer just an afterthought or suggestion. Our patient census continues to go up as more people see value in it. When we started, everyone thought this one oncologist was going to be a big obstacle. He interacted okay with me but did not talk to the nurses or social workers on the core team. Not anymore. Now he interacts with them like they are best friends, and all I hear is praises.

Box 1.5 shows the foundational role of communication in action via a successful organizational change campaign to improve patient outcomes (Wick et al., 2015).

BOX 1.5

FOUNDATIONAL ROLE OF COMMUNICATION IN ACTION

What: Johns Hopkins Hospital utilized a trust-based accountability model to improve patient-centered outcomes, experience, and value in colorectal surgery (Wick et al., 2015).

Who: Organizational members of all levels and areas of expertise, from the chief financial officer and senior vice president for patient safety and quality to frontline care providers

How: A meaning-centered approach to communication was enacted via a trust-based accountability model. Instead of approaching change as most organizations do (a) from a top-down approach with mandates from senior leadership, (b) with frontline employees trying to make meaningful changes without the support of senior leadership, or (c) without assembling an interdisciplinary project team, Johns Hopkins valued the expertise of each unit and highlighted the need to work collaboratively across the organization. This included a focus on the following:

1. Individual and unit responsibility, role clarity, and feedback
2. Capacity of all members to model safety related to their individual role
3. Providing members with the required resources, including time, to successfully consider, pilot test, and integrate new organizational processes

Results: The integration of new processes resulted in decreased lengths of stay and patients reported increased satisfaction with staff responsiveness, communication about medication, and pain management (p. 675). Moreover, over 90% of patients suggested that they would recommend the hospital to family and friends, which was more than a 10% increase from previous years.

Meaning-Centered Approach: The example in Box 1.5 illustrates a communicatively complex way of organizing and facilitating change in the healthcare setting. Stakeholders at all levels of the organization were integrated in meaningful ways, where members were empowered to share their expert opinions as the process unfolded. This illustrates that the organization took an audience-centered approach in letting the relevant experts weigh-in and guide aspects of the process that aligned with their individual expertise. Relatedly, this approach also illustrates active listening across the workgroup as members had to listen to understand the recommendations made by each area and thoughtfully consider how they would impact the process as a whole. The authors note that tweaks were made throughout the process, which demonstrates flexing communicatively in order to align individual roles, goals, and areas of expertise across multiple disciplines for the benefit of patient care.

Embracing a meaning-making approach is particularly helpful in environments of intense emotional labor like palliative care. This intensity compounded by communication challenges can lead to feelings of helplessness and higher rates of provider burnout. Some studies show up to 62% of palliative providers burn out (Kamal et al., 2016), and this remains the highest burn out rate of all healthcare specialties. Mnemonics such as RENEW (**R**ecognizing, **E**mbracing, **N**ourishing, **E**mbodying, and **W**eaving a New Response; Back, Rushton, Kaszniak, & Halifax, 2015) focus on processes to deal with this emotional intensity in caring environments. Models such as this one are strengthened when used in context with constructive intrapersonal communication practices such as mindfulness and effective team communication. The COMFORT model by Wittenberg-Lyles, Goldsmith, Richardson, Hallett, and Clark (2011) focuses on the nursing position in palliative care through **C**ommunication, **O**rientation and opportunity, **M**indful presence, **F**amily, **O**penings, **R**elating, and **T**eams. The oft-used model for nursing does nod to the nested position of the nurse in a team. The focus of this text is on the **T**—how to form and maintain healthy teams in palliative care. Exhibit 1.2 is an excerpt from a patient care coordination meeting (aka "rounds") where the team works to solve an issue for a patient.

The team in Exhibit 1.2 works well together for problem-solving. In this one situation, there are a number of factors that contribute to a problem that no one person is capable of solving on their own. It takes the team to understand and address each factor, including the following: the correct medication and its cost, the insurance issues, the nuances of a particular skilled nursing facility's admission practices, and the patient's social support system. The excerpt in Exhibit 1.2 is also an example of patient-centered care. This specific medication is what the patient needs, but the healthcare system is not built to easily help the patient. In less than 90 seconds, this team creates solution after solution. Most of the solutions have a flaw, and the team identifies that flaw and works out the next version of the solution. They arrive at a plan for how to solve this issue for this patient today that

EXHIBIT 1.2

MINI CASE STUDY: TEAM PROBLEM-SOLVING FOR A DIFFICULT DISCHARGE TO SKILLED NURSING FACILITY (SNF)

Dianne (APRN):	So Lila. Lila was supposed to go out today, but Kathy got a message from the doc that said they could not order a different med—Lila had a repeat sensitivity on her urine that was colonized; VRE was higher. So they're not okay with switching her to a less expensive antibiotic.
Kathy (PharmD):	Are the sensitivities back on that? On the second one?
Dianne:	Yeah, they are. She said the colonization was higher, and so they felt like if they put her on anything besides linezolid, she's not going to do well.
Kathy:	I did find out, though, that there is a program to help pay for linezolid. I can get my hands on the coupon, and it covers, like, $600.... the patient pays the first $15, and then it covers the next $600. If they… she does have insurance, right?
Miriam (Social Worker):	She does. Would we discharge her with that, then? Because how would you facilitate the SNF getting the drug for her?
Kathy:	Wait—if she goes to an SNF, do they not pay for her meds?
Miriam:	They do, but ... they won't pay for the linezolid.
Dianne:	So if you [Miriam] do her packet and send it with the packet and tell the SNF, "There's a coupon coming"—
Kathy:	I mean, that's what I want—I don't know the answer to that, if they can't or won't fill it.
Leslie (RN):	So does she have family? Could it be filled by somebody at a pharmacy, and then send it with the family?
Miriam:	It could be, but remember the admitting person at the SNF can be a mean lady.
Leslie:	Yeah, it would be difficult.
Kathy:	Okay, what if it was filled through our pharmacy?
Dianne:	That would work.
Kathy:	Could we just send the bottle with her, then?

Miriam:	Yeah. I mean, the same way you would send a patient's own medicine from here—yeah. I think that would work if it came from here.
Leslie:	Yeah. That would be optimal.
Kathy:	And then we'd need a script from the doctor and the doctor to fill something out on this coupon form. I think we can get it done today before the discharge.

matches the patient's need medically and financially while also circumventing some of the potential problems that occur when a patient is transferred from one facility to another. This interdisciplinary interaction exemplifies the importance of team-based palliative care. The team is efficient, collaborative, and creative in their problem-solving, and, most importantly, they achieve their goal of providing excellent care for this seriously ill patient.

Ambiguity in Systems and Teams: A Primary Challenge for Palliative Care

A primary reason palliative care communication is so challenging is due to the equivocal nature of the discipline. Equivocality is the degree to which a situation is ambiguous or given to more than one meaning. Working with patients and families with life-limiting and/or life-ending diagnoses introduces uncertainty at many levels.

- Many healthcare providers still view palliative care as a sign that patients or their healthcare providers have given up and failed. The road map for caring for a patient without an intent to cure is confusing if a provider feels that they have failed the patient.
- PCTs are constructed of numerous disciplines. While they may be united in their desire to care for patients and families at the end of life, their training and practices may be quite different and involve numerous unconscious defaults in perception and decision-making.
- A team of multiple disciplines is involved in the complex organization of a hospital, and that complex organization often must work with other complex organizations such as hospices that are not affiliated with the hospital, social welfare agencies, and insurance companies.
- Palliative care providers have difficulty finding people outside their workplace who understand their jobs. This limits their options for discussing work outside the small circle of their immediate colleagues. As one nurse

shared, "Nobody else understands this kind of work … You can't really talk to your family because they say 'That sounds really sad.' It's really not." Her pharmacist colleague agreed, saying that before she joined the PCT, "I thought our meetings would be sadder, dryer. They really aren't."

All of these factors add up to a complex personal and familial health situation cared for by a complex group of people housed in a complex organization that interfaces with a complex system of organizations. Add emotional labor to all of that complexity (Figure 1.1) and it is no wonder that palliative programs are on the rise due to need while simultaneously suffering due to burnout.

Given the intensity and vital nature of the challenge to improve PCT functioning through better communication, Weick's (1995) *Sensemaking in Organizations* framework is a helpful guide. Weick explains that organizations, and the teams and groups of which they are made, are really verbs rather than static nouns. Organizations are always organizing and thus may be better understood as active bodies rather than fully formed and unchanging things. If we consider hospitals and PCTs in this light, the model of organizing better fits the day-to-day work as well as the attempt to evolve healthcare past the model of the separation of disciplines working in silos. Weick's work on high-reliability organizations (2005) fits healthcare systems perfectly. High-reliability organizations are those that operate in complex, high-hazard domains for extended periods without serious accidents or catastrophic failures (Agency for Healthcare Research and Quality, 2019). These organizations maintain an environment of mindfulness through the following actions: preoccupation with failure, reluctance to simplify, sensitivity to operations, deference to expertise, and commitment to resilience (Weick & Sutcliffe, 2007).

Sutcliffe et al. (2004) talk about the latent flaws in the medical system that can lead to mishaps and oversights in patient care. These obstacles include complex and fragmented healthcare systems, faulty or nonexistent communication,

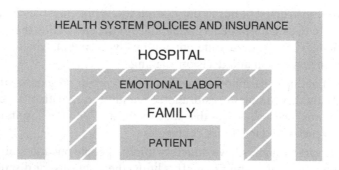

FIGURE 1.1 Emotional labor in palliative care.

hierarchies and power differences, fear of upward influence, role conflict and ambiguity, interpersonal power struggles, and team conflict. As teams work to overcome these obstacles, the following urges may be strong: to focus only on the positive, oversimplify relationships, ignore the larger context in which the team is embedded, revert to hierarchical decision-making, and decide that if the system does not work, it is the fault of an individual person. All of these leanings go against Weick's advice. Take the problem-solving case in Exhibit 1.2. This mini-case study shows team members working together in a somewhat ambiguous situation to discover a solution for a patient. They do not get angry when a member who is not in charge of prescribing has an idea, and they do not get frustrated when the initial ideas turn out to be unworkable. Their consistent engagement and focus on solving the problem results in a good solution for this patient.

Palliative Care Training and Education

As the need for palliative care remains strong, the number of palliative care fellowships and master's certificates continues to grow. While palliative specialists are needed, primary palliative education is also required to ensure that:

1. Patients have healthcare professionals who understand the need to offer a range of options including good pain management.
2. Physicians make referrals to PCTs when appropriate.

However, change comes slowly to all fields, and the 2014 IOM report notes that widespread adoption of timely referral to palliative care has been slow (IOM, 2014). While gains in clinical skills for seriously ill patient care are improving, understanding of palliative care is still deficient for many newly educated physicians. For example, a 2015 study of 176 hematology and oncology fellows found that 100% felt it was important to learn how to care for the dying, and, compared to an earlier survey, the number of fellows completing a palliative care rotation rose from 26% in 2005 to 44.9% in 2015 (Thomas et al., 2015). The study also found increasing competency in the following areas: pain management, informing patients of poor prognoses, and determining when to refer a patient to hospice. These increases in clinical skills are important for patient care. However, the study also found that "25% of fellows reported no explicit teaching on key palliative care skills such as assessing prognosis, conducting a family meeting to discuss treatment options, and referral to palliative care" (p. 749). These data remind us that while medical education continues to add to the skill base and awareness of physicians, there remains a need for better preparation of providers to work together at the interdisciplinary level and do the complex and vital work of palliative care on PCTs.

One way to approach this complex work is to reconsider how teams are constructed and their norms for working together. Across the professional practice of PCTs, conceptualizing teams as transdisciplinary rather than interdisciplinary points out a new way of functioning. In addition to drawing from multiple disciplines, transdisciplinarity "integrates natural, social and health sciences … and transcends their traditional boundaries" (Choi & Pak, 2006, p. 351). This text uses the term *interdisciplinary*. Although the use of *transdisciplinary* is gaining traction in organizations such as CAPC, it is not a widely used term at this time. For interdisciplinary and transdisciplinary teams, communication becomes even more vital for connecting and sharing information across disciplines. David Weissman, founding editor of the *Journal of Palliative Medicine*, notes that while ever-increasing demand for palliative care services and teams is good news, "the downside is that most teams I meet with are struggling, overwhelmed by work demands.… Faced with growing clinical demands, teams follow a predicable path, whereby they increase their clinical workload at the expense of data collection, education, quality improvement, and most importantly, team health" (2015, p. 204). Weissman finds that stressed teams tend to retreat to their silos and abandon even the appearance of relying on the other disciplines in their teams and thus violating "a foundational precept of palliative care" (2015, p. 204).

Weissman's observations concerning stressed teams retreating to silos is a process worthy of more study due to the growing reliance on teams in healthcare and particularly for PCTs. As hospitals and health systems move to form more PCTs to benefit patients and bottom lines, treating team formation as a simplistic process can easily backfire. Considerations such as professional identity, team identity, conflict styles, and organizational culture will all impact the success of a PCT.

An additional challenge for palliative care is that this care functions best as interdisciplinary teams, and that, too, is expertise in short supply. Healthcare providers often have interdisciplinary experience outside of a team-based workplace. For example, many clinicians in cancer care routinely work with social workers and chaplains as well as nurses and other healthcare providers (Eggly et al., 2009). Thus, while they have experience consulting other disciplines, they have less experiences thinking as a team and considering resources (human and budgetary) as a team. The ability to work competently in interdisciplinary settings goes beyond the ability to be a nice person with whom people like to work. Teams are complex, and PCTs must work in a context that is also complex on many levels including care of seriously ill patients and communication with patients and their families. These multilayered medical and interpersonal situations also take place in the complexity of hospital and health systems, which are affected by healthcare policy and financial concerns.

One way to describe palliative care environments for information and relationships is the concept of *equivocality*. Equivocal environments have many information and relational inputs. As palliative care adds multiple layers of organizational decision-making in an ever-changing policy environment, a very complex system emerges. Karl Weick (1995) coined the term *requisite variety* to explain that complex organizations require problem-solving ability that matches that level of complexity. This way of thinking about meaning making and equivocality in organizations is not unlike a differential diagnosis. To reach a diagnosis, healthcare providers consider the numerous possibilities based on the symptoms. Those symptoms are considered in the context of the patient's history, age, and environment, among other factors, and the conclusion is drawn about the most likely cause of the symptoms. The symptoms and patient history and everything else considered for the patient are like the equivocality in teams. Given the many informational inputs, a PCT meets the requisite variety because it assembles the range of knowledge and practice needed for the patient on one team. As the problems to be solved in palliative care range from medication decisions to family conflict to department-based conflict, the team will work best when communicatively competent healthcare professionals are prepared to be nimble in thought and practice as they help seriously ill patients and their families.

Palliative care involves numerous moving parts, and therefore, simply assembling a team of people who fit the disciplinary requirements for the team is unlikely to result in the characteristics of high-performing PCTs noted in Table 1.1. A 2018 study of primary PCTs in the United Kingdom found that the 2011 Gold Standards Framework, a well-researched and presented guide of the care of end-of-life patients and their families, fails to help teams perform better because while it tells them what to do, it does not help teams understand how to work together to achieve the stated goals (Hackett, Ziegler, Godfrey, Foy, & Bennett, 2018). As one physician on a high-performing PCT wondered, "How did we build a team that's been this high-functioning and successful? Divine intervention?" His question indicates that while high-performing teams are the result of conscientious communication and attention to team development, the process for achieving high-performing status may be hard to recognize and perform. This text will assist teams and organizations in discovering the necessary elements to help them form and maintain high-performing PCTs.

Given the call to meet a growing need for palliative care, it is tempting to believe that simply creating more PCTs is the answer. However, such teams must also be visible and supported in their hospitals. Patients get to PCTs through referrals, and thus, PCTs must not only work to be a great team but also work with other clinicians to get referrals. A 2018 study on the growth of the subspecialty of pediatric palliative care teams (PPCTs) found that the most persuasive element to convince clinicians to provide referrals was educating non-PPCT clinicians that one call/referral to the PPCT meant that the referring clinician was spared coordinating large groups of professionals for the patient's case. The PPCT was already organized to coordinate that care in conjunction with the referring physician (Verberne et al., 2018). This discovery led to an increase in referrals, and that increase was amplified when referring physicians reported that the quality of the patient's care increased due to the involvement of the PPCT. In other words, good press begets more interest and referrals and shows that the investment in forming and maintaining a high-performing PCT will likely continue to grow through referrals as the good news of the team spreads through the hospital and healthcare systems.

Conclusion

This chapter started by examining three truths of palliative care. Each chapter in the rest of the book takes on one of the big topics in PCT communication: PCT membership, forming and maintaining high-performing teams, team leadership, team meetings, occupational culture, and avoiding burnout through good self-care and the creation of a healthy team environment. Chapters include many reflections and experiences from those working in palliative care, and each chapter concludes with a few "Pearls From the Field" to guide your continued learning on developing and maintaining high-performing teams.

The need for PCTs will continue to grow. However, without a focus on intentional communication, team building, and relational maintenance, teams are likely to have high turnover rates. The high intensity of patient and family work in palliative care amplifies the stakes—if organizations and team leaders do not build a team that helps one another thrive through working together, the teams themselves become one more factor that adds to high burnout rates. This text is designed to provide workable solutions to challenges such as poor team design, siloing, and faulty communication. This focus allows groups of professions who are passionate about palliative care to grow into high-performing teams with a focus on patient care.

Ultimately, good palliative care is provided for patients and families through team-based care constructed from clinical expertise and skillful communication. When done well, PCTs do more than provide care and comfort for patients and families with serious illnesses. PCTs can offer emotional support, personal and occupational identity clarity, and organizational benefits to palliative care professionals. When the mission of the profession is to care for others in their time of great need, focus on building strong and sustainable PCTs is necessary.

PEARLS FROM THE FIELD: PROVIDER AND TEAM TAKEAWAYS

Takeaway 1: Palliative care is important work and palliative care teams are an excellent way to accomplish patient and family care.

The vital work of palliative care can be exhausting—patients and families dealing with serious illness and complex healthcare systems have many needs, and those needs can wear on even the most practiced palliative care provider. Utilizing PCTs is an efficient and effective way to provide great care while capitalizing on the expertise of numerous specialties on a single team. Each PCT member learns from and can lean on other team members, as they help patients and families navigate healthcare systems, physical and emotional experiences, spiritual questions, and the logistics of care. Great teams help team members do more than survive the difficulties of such work; they help them to thrive.

Takeaway 2: Effective communication is intentional and can be time-consuming but can prevent medical mishaps and destructive team conflict.

Communication is the oft-cited but seldom explored centerpiece of communication between patients and providers, patients and families, providers and families, and providers with one another. Making the effort to learn to recognize effective communication is a worthwhile investment for providers and for PCTs. A strong, healthy team has the benefit of multiple perspectives. They also have sufficient trust to question one another for the well-being of the patient without throwing the team into destructive conflict every time a decision or order is questioned. A healthy team expects input from team members, and that input can save the team from making medical mistakes in the care of seriously ill patients.

References

Agency for Healthcare Research and Quality. (2019). *Patient safety primer: High reliability.* Retrieved from https://psnet.ahrq.gov/primers/primer/31/High-Reliability

Atayee, R., & Edmonds, K. P. (2018). This is why we eat lunch together. *Journal of Palliative Care, 21*(10), 1386. doi:10.1098/jpm.2018.0274

Bachmann, C., Abramovitch, H., Barbu, C. G., Cavaco, A. M., Elorza, R. D., Haak, R., … Rosenbaum, M. (2013). A European consensus on learning objectives for a core communication curriculum in health care professions. *Patient Education and Counseling, 1*, 18–26. doi:10.1016/j.pec.2012.10.016

Back, A. L., Rushton, C. H., Kaszniak, A. W., & Halifax, J. S. (2015). "Why are we doing this?": Clinician helplessness in the face of suffering. *Journal of Palliative Medicine, 18*(1), 26–30. doi:10.1089/jpm.2014.0115

Billings, J. A. (2002). Vicissitudes of the clinician-patient relationship in end-of-life care: Recognizing the role for teams. *Journal of Palliative Medicine, 5*(2), 295–299. doi:10.1089/109662102753641296

Candrian, C. (2015). The cost of care. *Health Communication, 30*, 732–736. doi:10.1080/1 0410236.2014.930771

Center to Advance Palliative Care. (2018). *Serious illness quality alignment hub scorecard 2018.* Retrieved from https://www.capc.org/payers-policymakers/quality-alignment-hub/

Center to Advance Palliative Care. (2019a). *Making the case: Research in the field.* Retrieved from https://registry.capc.org/metrics-resources/research-in-the-field/

Center to Advance Palliative Care. (2019b). *Reaching the tipping point.* Retrieved from https://tippingpointchallenge.capc.org/

Centers for Disease Control and Prevention. (2019). *Chronic diseases in America.* Retrieved from https://www.cdc.gov/chronicdisease/resources/infographic/chronic-diseases .htm

Choi, B. C., & Pak, A. W. (2006). Multidisciplinarity, interdisciplinarity and transdisciplinarity in health research services, education and policy. *Clinical Investigation Medicine, 29*(6), 351–364.

Compton-Phillips, A., & Mohta, N. S. (2019, June 6). Care redesign survey: The power of palliative care. *NEJM Catalyst.* Retrieved from https://catalyst.nejm.org/power-palliative -end-of-life-care-program/

Davis, M. P., Temel, J. S., Balboni, T., & Glare, P. (2015). A review of the trials which examine early integration of outpatient and home palliative care for patients with serious illnesses. *Annals of Palliative Medicine 4*(3), 99–121. doi:10.3978/j.issn.2224-5820.2015.04.04

Dudley, N., Chapman, S., & Spetz, J. (2018). Community-based palliative care leaders perspectives on staffing, recruitment, and training. *Journal of Hospice & Palliative Nursing, 20*(2), 146–152. doi:10.1097/NJH.0000000000000419

Dumanovsky, T., Augustin, R., Rogers, M., Lettang, K., Meier, D. E., & Morrison, R. S. (2016). The growth of palliative care in U.S. hospitals: A status report. *Journal of Palliative Medicine, 19*(1), 8–15. doi:10.1089/jpm.2015.0351

Eggly, S. S., Albrecht, T. L., Kelly, K., Prigerson, H. G., Kennedy Sheldon, L., & Studts, J. (2009). The role of the clinician in cancer clinical communication. *Journal of Health Communication, 14*(Suppl. 1), 66–75. doi:10.1080/10810730902806778

Fulmer, T., Escobedo, M., Berman, A., Koren, M. J., Hernández, S., & Hult, A. (2018). Physicians' views on advance care planning and end-of-life care conversations. *Journal of the American Geriatrics Society, 66*, 1201–1205. doi:10.1111/jgs.15374

Hackett, J., Ziegler, L., Godfrey, M., Foy, R., & Bennett, M. I. (2018). Primary palliative care team perspectives on coordinating and managing people with advanced cancer in the community: A qualitative study. *BMC Family Practice, 19*, 177. doi:10.1186/s12875-018-0861-z

Hales, S., Zimmermann, C., & Robin G. (2010). Review: The quality of dying and death: A systematic review of measures. *Palliative Medicine, 24*(2), 127–144. doi:10.1177/ 0269216309351783

Imes, R. S., & Hester, J. (2015). *Unintended intentional community at work: Applying a new lens to guide the formation and maintenance of transdisciplinary teams.* Paper presented at the National Communication Association Annual Convention, Las Vegas.

Institute of Medicine. (2014). *Dying in America: Improving quality and honoring preferences near the end of life.* National Academy of Sciences. Retrieved from http://www .nationalacademies.org/hmd/Reports/2014/Dying-In-America-Improving -Quality-and-Honoring-Individual-Preferences-Near-the-End-of-Life.aspx

Jennings, T. (Producer). (2015). Being mortal [series episode]. *Frontline.* Boston, MA: PBS Broadcasting.

Kamal, A., Bull, J., Swetz, K., Wolf, S., Shanafelt, T., & Myers, E. (2017). Future of the palliative care workforce: A preview to an impending crisis. *The American Journal of Medicine, 130*(2), 113–114.

Kamal, A. H., Bull, J. H., Wolf, M. S., Swetz, K. M., Shanafelt, T. D., & Abernathty, A. P. (2016). Prevalence and predictors of burnout among hospice and palliative care clinicians in the U.S. *Journal of Pain and Symptom Management, 51*(4), 690–696. doi:10.1016/j.jpainsymman.2015.10.020

Kavalieratos, D., Corbelli, J., Zhang, D., Dionne-Odom, J. N., Ernecoff, N. C., Hanmer, J., … Schenker, Y. (2016). Association between palliative care and patient and caregiver outcomes: A systematic review and meta-analysis. *JAMA, 316*(20), 2104–2114. doi:10.1001/jama.2016.16840

Kerr, C. W., Tangeman, J. C., Rudra, C. B, Grant, P. C., Luckiewicz, D. L., Mylotte, K. M., … Serehali, A. M. (2014). Clinical impact of a home-based palliative care program: A hospice-private payer partnership. *Journal of Pain and Symptom Management, 48*(5), 883–892. doi:10.1016/j.jpainsymman.2014.02.003

Klarare, A., Hagelin, C. L., Fürst, C. J., & Fossum, B. (2013). Team interactions in specialized palliative care teams: A qualitative study. *Journal of Palliative Medicine, 16*(9), 1062–1069. doi:10.1089/jpm.2012.0622

Kousaie, K., & van Gunten, C. F. (2017). Models of palliative care team composition: Nurse practitioner-only versus interdisciplinary teams that include specialist physicians. *Journal of Palliative Medicine, 20*(12), 1313. doi:10.1089/jpm.2017.0380

Ledford, C., Canzona, M., Cafferty, L., & Kalish, V. (2016). Negotiating the equivocality of palliative care: A grounded theory of team communicative processes in inpatient medicine. *Health Communication, 31*(5), 1–8. doi:10.1080/10410236.2014.974134

Lingard, L., Whyte, S., & Regehr, G. (2009). *Safer surgery: Analysing behaviour in the operating theatre.* Surrey, UK: Ashgate Publishing.

Makary, M. A., & Daniel, M. (2016). Medical error—The third leading cause of death in the US. *BMJ, 353,* i2139.

May, P., Garrido, M. M., Cassel, J. B., Kelley, A. S., Meier, D. E., Normand, C., … Morrison, R. S. (2017). Cost analysis of a prospective multi-site cohort study of palliative care consultation teams for adults with advanced cancer: Where do cost-savings come from? *Palliative Medicine, 31*(4), 378–386. doi:10.1177/0269216317690098

May, P., Normand, C., Cassell, J. B., Del Fabbro, E., Fine, R. L., Menz, R., … Morrison, R. S. (2018). Economics of palliative care for hospitalized adults with serious illness: A meta-analysis. *JAMA Internal Medicine, 178*(6), 820–829. doi:10.1001/jamainternmed.2018.0750

McCarthy, I. M., Robinson, C., Huq, S., Philastre, M., & Fine, R. L. (2015). Cost savings from palliative care teams and guidance for a financially viable palliative care program. *Health Services Research, 50*(1), 217–236. doi:10.1111/1475-6773.12203

Meier, D. (2019). "The Future of Palliative Care: A Podcast with Diane Meier" GeriPal - A Geriatrics and Palliative Care Podcast. Retrieved from https://www.geripal.org/p/geripal-podcast.html

Meier, D. E., Back, A. L., Berman, A., Block, S. D., Corrigan, J. M., & Morrison, R. S. (2017). A national strategy for palliative care. *Health Affairs, 26*(7), 1265–1273. doi:10.1377/hlthaff.2017.0164

National Consensus Project. (2018). *Clinical practice guidelines for quality palliative care* (4th ed.). Richmond, VA: National Coalition for Hospice and Palliative Care. Retrieved from https://www.nationalcoalitionhpc.org/ncp

National Palliative Care Registry. (2017). *Metrics and resources.* Retrieved from https://registry.capc.org/metrics-resources/

Nussbaum, J. F., & Fisher, C. L. (2009). A communication model for the competent delivery of geriatric medicine. *Journal of Language and Social Psychology, 28*(2), 190–208. doi:10.1177/0261927X08330609

Omilion-Hodges, L. M., & Baker, C. R. (2017). Communicating leader-member relationship quality: The development of leader communication exchange scales to measure relationship building and maintenance through the exchange of communication-based goods. *International Journal of Business Communication, 54*(2), 115–145. doi:10.1177/2329488416687052

Parker, J. (2019, April 4). Palliative care could cut health care costs by $103B. *Hospice News.* Retrieved from https://hospicenews.com/2019/04/04/palliative-care-could-cut-health-care-costs-by-103-billion/

Quill, T. E., & Abernathy, A. P. (2013). Generalist plus specialist palliative care--Creating a more sustainable model. *The New England Journal of Medicine, 368*(13), 1173–1175. doi:10.1056/NEJMp1215620

Scharf, B. F., Geist Martin, P., Cosgriff-Hernandez, K.-K., & Moore, J. (2012). Trailblazing healthcare: Institutionalizing and integrating complementary medicine. *Patient Education and Counseling 89*, 434–438. doi:10.1016/j.pec.2012.03.006

Smith, T. J., Temin, S., Alesi, E. R., Abernethy, A. P., Balboni, T. A., Basch, E. M., . . . Von Roenn, J. H. (2012). American Society of Clinical Oncology provisional clinical opinion: The integration of palliative care into standard oncology care. *Journal of Clinical Oncology, 30*(8), 880–7. doi:10.1200/JCO.2011.38.5161

Spetz, J., Dudly, N., Trupin, L., Rogers, M., Meier, D. E., & Dumanovsky, T. (2016). Few hospital palliative care programs meet national staffing recommendations. *Health Affairs, 35*(9), 1690–1697. doi:10.1377/hlthaff.2016.0113

Sutcliffe, K. M., Lewton, E., & Rosenthal, M. M. (2004). Communication failures: An insidious contributor to medical mishaps. *Academic Medicine, 79*(2), 186–194. doi:10.1097/00001888-200402000-00019

Thomas, R. A., Curley, B., Wen, S., Zhang, J., Abrahman, J., & Moss, A. H. (2015). Palliative care training during fellowship: A national survey of U.S. Hematology and Oncology Fellows. *Journal of Palliative Medicine, 18*(9), 747–751. doi:10.1089/jpm.2015.0035

Verberne, L. M., Kars, M. C., Schepers, S. A., Schouten-van Meeteren, A. Y. N., Grootenhuis, M. A., & van Delden, J. J. M. (2018). Barriers and facilitators to the implementation of a paediatric palliative care team. *BMC Palliative Care, 17*(1), 23. doi:10.1186/s12904-018-0274-8

Watson, B. M., Heatley, M. L., Gallois, C., & Kruske, S. (2016). The importance of effective communication in interprofessional practice: Perspectives of maternity clinicians. *Health Communication, 31*(4), 400–407. doi:10.1080/10410236.2014.9609222

Weick, K. (1995). *Sensemaking in organizations.* Thousand Oaks, CA: Sage.

Weick, K. (2005). Managing the unexpected: Complexity as distributed sensemaking. In R. R. McDaniel & D. J. Dreibe (Eds.), *Uncertain and surprise in complex systems: Question on working with the unexpected* (pp. 51–78). Berlin: Springer-Verlag.

Weick, K. E., & Sutcliffe, K. M. (2007). *Managing the unexpected: Resilient performance in an age of uncertainty.* San Francisco, CA: Jossey-Bass.

Weissman, D. E. (2015). Improving care during a time of crisis: The evolving role of specialty palliative care teams. *Journal of Palliative Medicine, 18*(3), 204–207. doi:10.1089/jpm.2015.1014

Wick, E. C., Galante, D. J., Hobson, D. B., Benson, A. R., Lee, K. H. K., ...Wu, C. L. (2015). Organizational culture changes result in improvement in patient-centered outcomes:

Implementation of an integrated recovery pathway for surgical patients. *Journal of the American College of Surgeons, 221*(3), 669–677. doi:10.1016/j.jamcollsurg.2015.05.008

Wittenberg-Lyles, E., Goldsmith, J., Richardson, B., Hallett, J. S., & Clark, R. (2012). The practical nurse: A case for COMFORT communication training. *American Journal of Hospital and Palliative Medicine, 30*(2), 162–166. doi:10.1177/1049909112446848

World Health Organization. (2017). *WHO definition of palliative care.* Retrieved from http://www.who.int/cancer/palliative/definition/en/

CHAPTER 2

WHO ARE THE PLAYERS? EXPLORING THE TYPES OF PALLIATIVE CARE PROVIDERS

Introduction

At its core, palliative care tends to human suffering. It would be a mistake to define suffering as merely a physical complaint such as pain. Cicely Saunders, widely known for her founding role in the modern hospice movement, expanded the understanding of "total pain" as the suffering that encompasses all of a person's physical, psychological, social, spiritual, and practical struggles (Richmond, 2005). According to Ferrell and Coyle (2008), suffering is distress that is related to pain, discomfort, grief, loss, helplessness, inability to cope, isolation, and loss of meaning. Effective management of suffering requires interdisciplinary team members who are uniquely prepared not only to recognize and treat a symptom but also to understand and address the factors affecting the person living with the symptom (Sumser, Leimena, & Altilio, 2019).

Negative Palliative Care Experience

Patient Perspective: Sometimes it feels like I'm just another number on the 0 to 10 pain scale. I tell the nurse that I hurt all over, and she gets me the pain medicine the doctor ordered but my mind is going in circles—Why did this happen to me? Who is going to take care of my dog? How am I going to pay for this? The medicine sort of helps but, mostly, I think it lets me zone out for a little bit. I still don't know what to do about the other questions.

Positive Palliative Care Experience

Family Perspective: I can't imagine going through this without the palliative care team. The doctor spent a long time really trying to understand my dad's pain, and she picked a medicine that really seems to work. We were completely lost and trying

---

A podcast to accompany this chapter is available with online access of this title. Please see the instructions on the first page of the book for details on how to access and go to Chapter 2.

TABLE 2.1 **Domains of Care**

DOMAIN	ASPECT OF CARE	FOCUS
1	Structure and processes of care	Composition of an interdisciplinary team, including professional qualifications, education, training, and support needed to deliver optimal patient- and family-centered care. Elements of systems and processes, the palliative care assessment, and care plan across settings
2	Physical aspects of care	Relief of physical symptoms (e.g., pain, dyspnea, constipation) and improving or maintaining functional status
3	Psychological and psychiatric aspects of care	Common psychological issues (e.g., emotional distress, anxiety, depression, delirium, substance abuse disorder) and complex psychiatric issues
4	Social aspects of care	Patient/family structure and support systems, community resources, care environments, and the impact of social and financial barriers to care
5	Spiritual, religious, and existential aspects of care	Spiritual background, preferences, and related beliefs, values, rituals, and practices. Meaning seeking, purpose, and transcendence of illness
6	Cultural aspects of care	Cultural beliefs, values, traditional practices, language, and communication preferences related to race, ethnicity, gender identity and expression, sexual orientation, immigration and refugee status, social class, religion, spirituality, physical appearance, and abilities
7	Care of the patient nearing the end of life	Signs and symptoms of the dying process and communication with family about imminent death, transitions of care, and grief and bereavement
8	Ethical and legal aspects of care	Advanced care planning and documentation, surrogate decision-making, ethical and legal principles

SOURCE: National Consensus Project for Hospice and Palliative Care. (2018). *Clinical practice guidelines for quality palliative care* (4th ed.). Richmond, VA: National Coalition for Hospice and Palliative Care. Retrieved from https://www.nationalcoalitionhpc.org/ncp/

to figure out what we were going to do after leaving the hospital, but the social worker has advocated for us every step of the way. My dad wouldn't say what he and the chaplain talked about the other day but he's seemed so relaxed since then— for the first time, he's been telling us all these wonderful stories from his childhood.

Domains of Care

Patients and families dealing with serious illness require a range of professional services. To this point, the National Consensus Project (NCP) Clinical Practice Guidelines for Quality Palliative Care, Fourth Edition (2018), identifies domains that include physical, psychological, psychiatric, social, cultural, spiritual, religious, and existential aspects of care (see Table 2.1).

Disciplines are rooted in particular domains: medicine and nursing in the physical domain, social work in the psychological and social domains, and chaplaincy in the spiritual domain. Like the human experience of serious illness, however, these domains do not stand alone in silos waiting for a straightforward response from an individual team member who is uniquely prepared to address a single source of suffering. Professional training and background bring particular strengths to specific aspects of care, but these domains overlap and interplay with each other, calling upon interdisciplinary team members to bring their own professional expertise to each domain.

According to Coyle (1997, p. 266), the idea "that the ability to perform such a comprehensive assessment as well as institute the necessary, ongoing interventions and monitoring, could lie within the purview of one profession … is unrealistic." Unlike Cicely Saunders, who was trained as a nurse, a social worker (SW), and a physician, most clinicians cannot be expected to expertly assess and manage all aspects of care alone. This work takes a village (Figure 2.1).

Who Are the Palliative Care Specialists?

Palliative care specialists should have formal training in palliative care beyond basic competency and may be certified in their discipline. The recently revised NCP Guidelines (2018) specifically identify the following disciplines as core members of specialty palliative care teams (PCTs): physicians, nurses, advanced practice providers, social workers, chaplains, and clinical pharmacists. This chapter focuses on these disciplines.

Though palliative care programs may not require board certification for all PCT members, per the NCP Guidelines (2018), all should demonstrate specialty-level competency. As a relatively new subspecialty, formal training programs and board certification for palliative care clinicians have only recently become

A CASE STUDY: THROUGH DIFFERENT LENSES

The palliative care service was consulted to assist with goals of care for a family struggling to decide whether to place a PEG (percutaneous endoscopic gastrostomy) tube in an 87-year old African American woman with advanced dementia who was hospitalized for aspiration pneumonia. Team members see the same situation through different lenses and approach care comprehensively together.

REGISTERED NURSE
STRUCTURE OF CARE, PHYSICAL DOMAIN

I was the first member of the team to meet the family, so I introduced the idea of palliative care and arranged a family meeting when it was clear that everyone needed to come together on this decision. Afterward, they were still really struggling to imagine what tube feedings through a PEG tube would be like. I used pictures to show them what a PEG tube looks like and how you actually give the feedings. I also talked with them about how to offer careful handfeeding as an alternative to tube feeding and offered to coordinate a visit with the speech pathologist to learn more.

PHARMACIST — PHYSICAL DOMAIN

I reviewed this patient's medication list and identified a medication that might be contributing to her delirium, which might have contributed to her inability to effectively swallow in recent weeks. If she was able to be more alert, she might be able to more safely eat the food her family so lovingly wanted to feed her.

SAME PATIENT • FAMILY DIFFERENT LENSES

PHYSICIAN — PHYSICAL DOMAIN

I diagnosed the stage of the patient's dementia based on the family's report of her baseline function over the past few months. I helped them understand her prognosis and the implications of the treatment options they were offered. They were very worried about her shortness of breath with the pneumonia, so I made recommendations to treat that symptom.

CHAPLAIN — CULTURAL, SPIRITUAL DOMAINS

I tended to their grief at the recent loss of a loved one and the anticipatory grief for the patient who was nearing the terminal stage of her disease. They worried that God would judge them for "starving" the patient if they decided to forgo the feeding tube. I addressed their spiritual distress, had prayer with them, and offered to reach out to their much loved pastor for spiritual guidance. I also had a listening ear for their family culture around caring for one's elderly at home at all costs. Rather than try to talk them out of a deeply held value, I challenged my team to help this family find ways to make it work for them to care for this patient at home.

SOCIAL WORKER — PSYCHOLOGICAL, SOCIAL, ETHICAL/LEGAL DOMAINS

Even though this patient never completed advanced directives, I helped them understand the process for surrogate decision-making within the structure and dynamics of their family. I also addressed some of their logistical concerns and emotional distress about who would stay with this patient at home following the recent sudden death of her sister who had been her primary caregiver. The family had promised her they would never "throw her away into a nursing home," but no one was in a financial position to give up their job to care for her at home.

FIGURE 2.1 A case study: Through different lenses.

available (if at all, for some disciplines). Many of the most experienced palliative care clinicians learned "on the job" and have gone on to identify core competencies and to create the training and certification opportunities for the next generation of clinicians (Dahlin, Coyne, & Ferrell, 2016). Many palliative care clinicians received formal training in other areas such as family medicine, geriatrics, or oncology, and they bring this expertise to their palliative care practice as well.

Palliative care physicians can seek board certification through the American Board of Medical Specialties, which, starting in 2013, requires completion of an accredited Hospice and Palliative Medicine fellowship program. Nurses (RNs and APRNs) and social workers who have the required number of hours of supervised experience in hospice or palliative care are eligible for board examinations for their disciplines. Board-certified chaplains can earn advanced certification in palliative care and hospice either through written or interview application or completion of an action/reflection workshop. No palliative care certification for pharmacists currently exists, though, but like all clinicians who are interested in formal specialization training, they are eligible for interdisciplinary master's-level degrees and certificate programs in palliative care.

Physician Role

Physicians will have completed either an allopathic (MD) or osteopathic (DO) medical degree and a specialized residency program with the option of subspecialty fellowship training. A growing number of physicians have achieved specialty certification in hospice and palliative medicine in the past decade with the majority of primary board certification coming from internal medicine and family medicine (American Academy of Hospice and Palliative Medicine [AAHPM], 2019).

The physician role on the PCT is centered around the physical aspects of care, focused on the diagnosis and management of difficult pain and symptoms, and the clinical judgment around communication on prognostication and treatment options. Physicians are responsible for developing individualized treatment plans by aligning patient and family preferences and wishes with the prognosis and treatment options offered by the primary medical team. While physicians often provide direct patient care, they may also be involved with collaboration or (depending on state law) oversight of other team members who practice within the physical domain. Physician involvement in some patient care may be offered through ongoing, day-to-day clinical guidance and recommendations to fellow PCT members. Physicians may also provide on-call coverage.

BOX 2.1

A PHYSICIAN REFLECTS: PERSPECTIVE ON ROLES

I have been practicing medicine for years, and working as a team has made me the happiest I have ever been in my career. As a physician, there is this expectation that you are the sole person to make clinical decisions and that everyone else is around to follow your orders. It is a lot of power, but it is also very isolating and, frankly, kind of scary at times to believe yourself to be solely responsible for fixing everything in a really complicated and emotional situation. When you work closely with a team, you start to see all these things you didn't even know you didn't know. I have tried to be cognizant of my status as a physician in a healthcare system that tends to be pretty hierarchical. What I have learned is that by letting myself be a little vulnerable and work within a team, I have become a better physician and colleague.

Like other disciplines, participation in team meetings and patient coordination care meetings, also known as rounds, is important in order to understand and address the full spectrum of physical, emotional, and spiritual suffering. Physicians may also be called to communicate directly with physicians from other medical specialties in order to break down communication barriers related to hierarchical behaviors outside the PCT. For example, an attending physician in cardiology may insist on talking to a palliative care physician, not an APRN. However, during the meeting the palliative care physician may acknowledge that the treatment plan or proposed solution was offered by the APRN (or other team member). This allows the physician to forge a collaborative relationship for future referrals while also honoring individual team members and demonstrating the strength of the PCT. In Box 2.1, a physician reflects on the role.

Advanced Practice Provider Role

The term advanced practice providers (APPs) refers to physician assistants (PAs) and advanced practice registered nurses (APRNs). PAs are educated at the master's level and must pass a national certification exam and acquire state licensure. PAs can complete interdisciplinary postgraduate training programs in palliative care and participate in their own professional organization, the Physician Assistants in Hospice and Palliative Medicine (PAHPM); however, a palliative care specialty certification is not currently available for PAs.

The Consensus Model for APRN Regulation, Licensure, Certification, and Education Model (2008) provides guidance for states to adopt uniform regulations for APRN roles. Though variation exists between states, the model identifies the following master's or doctoral level APRN roles:

- Certified nurse practitioner (CNP)
- Clinical nurse specialist (CNS)
- Certified nurse midwife (CNM)
- Certified registered nurse anesthetist (CRNA)

Most palliative care APRNs are CNPs and CNSs, although CRNAs and CNMs may practice within areas of pain management and perinatal palliative care. APRNs are educated in one of six specific populations: family, adult/gerontology, neonatal, pediatrics, women's health, or psychiatric/mental health. APRNs are certified by an exam measuring competency in those specific patient populations. Specialty certification, such as ACHPN (Advanced Certified Hospice and Palliative Care Nurse), is not required to practice palliative care but is encouraged. The Competencies for the Hospice and Palliative Advanced Practice Nurse (Dahlin, 2014) outline the intellectual, interpersonal, technical, and moral competencies required for specialty-level care.

Depending on state laws governing practice, APPs provide direct patient care, including prescribing medications and diagnostic testing, either independently or with physician oversight to expand patient access to expert-level management of difficult pain and symptoms, prognostication, and communication

BOX 2.2

AN ADVANCED PRACTICE PROVIDER REFLECTS: PERSPECTIVE ON ROLES

I'm at my best and happiest when I can practice patient care to the full scope of my training while still knowing that my physician colleagues are at my fingertips for support and guidance. I always know they have my back and they never make me feel dumb when I ask for help with something like a symptom that is difficult to manage. They ask for my help, too, so it is really collaborative and safe. Since we are not all wrapped up in ego, I don't feel personally offended if a patient or another doctor wants to deal with a physician rather than an APRN. I know they will affirm my role in the case anyway. I see other APRNs around the hospital who seem to have been hired just to do their physician's scut work—they are actually called "physician extenders." On this team, I'm valued for my clinical expertise. This professional regard also gives me the confidence to mentor other staff around the hospital.

with patients, families, and the healthcare team regarding complex medical decision-making. APPs may also complete Practitioner Orders for Life Sustaining Treatment (POLST) or other code status documentation and provide on-call coverage.

In addition to the clinical focus of providing direct care to patients and families, APRNs are called upon to influence healthcare outcomes in populations, organizations, and health policy (American Association of Colleges of Nursing [AACN], 2004). APRNs may serve in a "dual consultant" role. In the medical model, APRNs provide expert palliative care directed at the patient and family level. In the nursing model, APRNs provide coaching and mentoring to other clinicians who provide palliative care (Ferrell & Paice, 2019). In Box 2.2, an APP reflects on the role.

Registered Nurse Role

Registered nurses (RNs) are state-licensed and may have completed a diploma program or associate's or bachelor's degree; however, most hospitals require a bachelor's degree. The American Nurses' Association (ANA, 2016) has defined the nursing role in the care of seriously ill patients to (a) include the duty to educate patients and families about end-of-life issues, (b) encourage discussion of preferences, (c) communicate relevant information to the care team, and (d) advocate for patients. Palliative care nursing practice involves expert-level "whole-person" care that includes assessment and management of symptoms, support across settings, collaboration with other members of the care team, and advocacy (Johnston & Smith, 2006).

RNs may serve in a number of capacities on a PCT. While they may provide direct patient care, they also serve as care coordinators, advocates, and educators. RNs are trained to assess the cultural and literacy needs of patients and families to provide effective teaching and understanding of the plan across care transitions.

RNs are well suited for serving as experts in the NCPG Domain 1—Structure and Processes of Care (NCP, 2018). With strong clinical understanding and expertise in collaboration, RNs may serve as "the hub of the wheel," promoting optimal communication among the team and with patients and families. This role may be realized through handling triage, taking on the role of information gathering for new consultations, and possibly, to be the first face the patient sees from the PCT. RNs may also provide follow-up visits for lower acuity patients, ensuring the PCT remains engaged with the patient and the primary care team, identifying changes in condition that might warrant re-engagement with the physician or APP. RNs can also ensure quality measures are consistently met by

BOX 2.3

A REGISTERED NURSE REFLECTS: PERSPECTIVE ON ROLES

As a nurse, I feel like I'm the glue that holds this whole operation together. As patient needs ebb and flow from hour to hour, there has to be a structure in place to make sure everyone gets great care and my team doesn't fall apart. I'm the one who knows what is going on with everyone on the team, and I have a good idea of what's happening with patients and families too, so I can triage calls, handle new consults effectively, and make sure patients have safe care transitions. So, in that way, maybe I'm more like air traffic control. When patients have long hospitalizations, families will get to know me as I do some of the follow-up visits, so the physicians and APRNs can see new patients. Patients learn to trust me as an advocate and a "holder of their story" even on days when things are stable.

the PCT and to teach and mentor staff. The Institute of Medicine's (IOM) Future of Nursing recommends that nurses be allowed to practice to the full extent of their education and training and should be regarded as full partners with physicians and other health professionals (IOM, 2011). In Box 2.3, an RN reflects on the role.

Social Worker Role

Social workers (SW) are the team experts on psychological and social aspects of care. SWs may be primarily responsible for the identification and management of psychosocial, financial, and logistical barriers to care; the assessment of adaptation to illness; anticipatory grief and coping strategies; supportive counseling for depression and anxiety; and evaluation of family and community support, home safety, and caregiver fatigue. SWs participating in care planning promote seamless care transitions, ensuring that patient and family goals and wishes are communicated across settings (Head, Peters, Middleton, Friedman, & Guman, 2019; Otis-Green, Sidhu, Del Ferraro, & Ferrell, 2014; Stein, Cagle, & Christ, 2017).

Palliative care specialty SW is an emerging role. In some institutions, there may be a misconception that all SWs, as clinical experts in psychosocial care, have the training and skills required to provide expert-level care to seriously ill patients and their families. In reality, not all SWs have had specialty palliative care training. Also, institutions assign and prioritize the role of discharge planning, which,

BOX 2.4

A SOCIAL WORKER REFLECTS: PERSPECTIVE ON ROLES

A common reason for referral to our palliative care service is to "clarify goals of care." On its face, it might seem like this is squarely in the purview of one of our medical people. You know—communicate the prognosis and identify treatment options that are aligned with a patient's wishes. In the end, though, you have to think about the family structure, how well they're coping, if they have the means to care for the patient in the way they would like, and whether anxiety is driving decision-making. A plan made in isolation of all this might sound really straightforward but, unless a family has good resources and bountiful emotional resilience, the whole thing can fall apart. You have to meet families where they are and help them make decisions within the context of their own lives. I bring that perspective to the table.

due to staffing pressures, may make it impossible for skilled primary SWs to focus on aspects of care that are unique to seriously ill patients, even if they would like to provide this care. For these reasons, tension between palliative care specialty SWs and primary/unit-based SWs may exist (Altilio & Otis-Green, 2011).

Benefits and burdens will emerge when a palliative care program and social work department decide that the palliative care SW will routinely "take over" all palliative care cases, including sole responsibility for discharge planning. Having the palliative care SW tend to all aspects of psychosocial and transitions of care may result in highly comprehensive and seamless patient care, but palliative care SW resources can become too stretched as referral volume grows. Therefore, sharing these responsibilities with the team may be advantageous.

Sharing patients requires a high level of communication and collaboration, which may be difficult when palliative care patients are scattered across the hospital under the care of multiple teams. Ideally, primary and palliative care SWs are able to practice collaboratively, honoring the importance of both roles whether deciding to work together on a particular case or determining that only one SW is needed. According to Sumser et al. (2019, p. 21), "The specialty palliative SW role is designed for flexibility and fluidity to respond and partner with the [primary] social worker in enriching clinical assessment, patient-family biopsychosocial care, family meetings, and psychosocial support for medical decision-making." In Box 2.4, a social worker reflects on the role.

An accompanying video, Right Care at the Right Time, presenting a social worker's perspective from Marjorie Rentz, may be accessed at connect.springerpub.com/content/book/978-0-8261-5806-2/ch02.

Chaplain Role

Chaplaincy preparation involves theological education, a master's in divinity (MDiv) or equivalent, ordination and endorsement by a faith group, and completion of four units of Clinical Pastoral Education (CPE). The units that comprise CPE include the following:

- Theory of pastoral care
- Identity and conduct
- Pastoral and professional competencies

According to a recent survey of palliative care chaplaincy in the United States (Jeuland, Fitchett, Schulman-Green, & Kapo, 2017), most palliative care chaplains (70%) are board-certified chaplains (BCCs).

Distinct from clergy who are appointed by and serve through the perspective of a particular denomination, interfaith chaplains help patients and families explore their own spirituality or existential meaning to cope with a serious illness whatever the faith tradition (or in cases where the patient does not identify with a particular faith). Indeed, the Association of Professional Chaplains' Code of Ethics prohibits chaplains from proselytizing or imposing their own beliefs on those receiving their care (2000).

A primary role of palliative care chaplains is spiritual care, which is informed by a spiritual history and spiritual assessment. According to a consensus report on improving the quality of spiritual care as a dimension of palliative care (Puchalski et al., 2009), a spiritual history is a structured interview to better understand a patient's spiritual needs and resources and can be conducted by non-chaplain PCT members. A spiritual assessment, however, is a more in-depth process of listening to a patient's story as it unfolds that may reveal concerns about hopes and fears, meaning, purpose, beliefs about the afterlife, guilt, forgiveness, and life completion tasks. A spiritual assessment is best conducted by a chaplain and should include a spiritual care plan with expected outcomes that are communicated to the healthcare team. According to Jeuland et al. (2017), palliative care chaplain visits often include chaplain craft (i.e., building relationship, providing ritual support, introducing spiritual care, and connecting patients with communities of faith), attending to death and dying, addressing goals of care, and tending to spiritual and existential distress.

Palliative care chaplains serve as educators on the role of the chaplain, religious practices, ethics, and advanced care planning. According to Abu-Ras (2011), as they are trained to understand how family cultures affect spiritual beliefs and practices, chaplains may establish expertise as "cultural brokers" who can navigate issues related to culture and religion that may be barriers to good communication. They

BOX 2.5

A CHAPLAIN REFLECTS: PERSPECTIVE ON ROLES

Our physician and pharmacist were really struggling to get hold of the nausea of a young patient with gastric cancer. We had tried a whole list of different medications, but nothing seemed to help. The nurses were so distressed watching her cry and wretch. When I had first met her, she declined my visit, saying she was not a "religious person." During rounds, we decided to offer another visit. She accepted this time, and I just sat with her, bearing witness to her suffering. Eventually, she was able to tell me that, ever since her cancer came back, it was like she could feel it growing in her stomach. It was not so much that it hurt as what it meant—that she was going to die too young, missing out on so much. She said it was like being lost at sea during a storm. Together, we came up with an image of calming waters with a lighthouse on the horizon that she could envision while doing breathing exercises. She still needed nausea medicine, but having this tool helped her regain some control.

may serve as translators among patients, families, and the healthcare team and encourage accommodation of people from various faiths and cultures. Also, through informal interactions, formal debriefing, or the facilitation of self-care activities and ritual, chaplains provide support to staff suffering from cumulative grief, moral distress, or vicarious trauma (Perez, 2015). In Box 2.5, a chaplain reflects on the role.

Pharmacist Role

Traditionally, the "core" PCT has included physicians, nurses, APPs, SWs, and chaplains with acknowledgment of the contributions of other professionals, which might include nutritionists, physical and occupational therapists, speech pathologists, and so forth. Increasingly, clinical pharmacists with special interest and training in palliative care are identified as important members of the team (Herndon et al., 2016). According to Pruskowski, Arnold, and Skeldar (2017), benefits of incorporating a palliative care pharmacist into the team include:

1. Improved pain and symptom management through expert-level understanding of pharmacology
2. Goal-concordant, patient-centered medication regimens
3. Enhanced coordination across care settings

BOX 2.6

A PHARMACIST REFLECTS: PERSPECTIVE ON ROLES

The palliative care team was involved in a left ventricular assist device (LVAD) workup and found an area of conflict that I was able to help resolve. The LVAD team felt that the patient was a good candidate for an LVAD, and the patient, in a general sense, agreed with the plan. The sticking point was that the patient was taking a bunch of supplements that the team did not know much about and the patient was *very* attached to. The team and the patient were at a complete impasse over this, so I sat down with the patient and his supplements and went through his rationale for each one. It turns out that he had some specific cultural reasons for taking them. When the team told him he had to stop taking them in order to safely get an LVAD, he had an emotional reaction. To him, it felt like a loss of control in an already scary situation. I researched all of the supplements and helped negotiate a safe compromise between the patient and the team.

The American Society of Health-System Pharmacists (ASHP) Guidelines on the Pharmacist's Role in Palliative and Hospice Care (2016) outlines essential and desirable roles and specialty-practice activities. Essential roles include direct patient care through the optimization of symptom medication regimens, medication order review and reconciliation, education and medication counseling for patients and families, and administrative involvement in safe use of medication in the treatment of pain and symptoms. Desirable roles include expanded involvement in patient care through direct, goal-directed pain and symptom assessment and management, development of educational opportunities for pharmacy students, contribution to scholarship through research and speaking, and practice and team leadership through policy and guideline development.

As the "resident experts" of pharmacology, the palliative care pharmacist's role resides primarily in the physical domain. Like other members of the interdisciplinary team, pharmacists who are able to integrate psychosocial and cultural aspects of care into the development of medication regimens are best positioned to facilitate improved physical outcomes. Also, pharmacists are well positioned to assist with the social domain of care (see Table 2.1) related to acquisition of medications and coordination during transitions of care. In Box 2.6, a pharmacist reflects on the role.

Leadership Role

Leadership on a PCT may range from formal to informal, often depending upon the maturity and size of the program. Newer, smaller teams often have more of an informal leadership structure where the team member with the most seniority or experience serves as the clinical and operational leader (often without commensurate title) and reports to an administrative leader(s). In this scenario, the administrative leader is minimally involved in day-to-day processes but may be appointed to oversee the team as a formality (Dahlin & Coyne, 2019). Informal clinical leaders are often APRNs, RNs, or SWs—sometimes chaplains or pharmacists—with physicians more likely to be titled as leaders. A culture of shared leadership across disciplines is critical for the success of a growing palliative program, which is achieved through shared responsibility for a common mission and vision, a collaborative team structure and care processes, and the ability to innovate and anticipate change.

In order to grow and function well, larger more mature teams require a clear organizational structure and, possibly, more direct administrative leadership along with clinical leadership to manage the implementation of programmatic processes. Ideally, team members report (at least indirectly) to an administrative leader who manages personnel, budgets, operational processes, and business planning and a clinical leader(s) who directs staff training and competencies, clinical processes, and referral relationships.

BOX 2.7

AN ADMINISTRATIVE LEADER REFLECTS: PERSPECTIVE ON ROLES

I came to the team a little later when the team was able to organize under a single management structure. It was a little humbling, at first, to "lead" a group of such highly skilled clinicians, but I have been able to bring management expertise to be able to help them get their operational needs met and to grow. I work closely with the team's clinical leaders. We problem-solve and make decisions together about hiring and the direction of the program. There is a great deal of trust among us, so it is safe to knock around ideas. We do not always agree, but in the end, we can speak as one voice to the rest of the team.

Administrative and clinical leaders are jointly responsible for:

1. Program alignment with the organization's goals
2. Integration into the care system
3. Continuous performance improvement
4. Innovation and conflict management
5. Awareness of external issues around care and payment models
6. Professional development of both clinical and administrative staff

Joint leadership requires a high level of professional respect, trust, and communication (Frieman & Nowicki, 2019). An expanded discussion of leadership on PCTs can be found in Chapter 4, Leading Palliative Care Teams. In Box 2.7, an administrative leader reflects on the role.

Role Clarity

Ideally, the skills and expertise of all disciplines on a PCT will be integrated into a patient's plan of care, with team members assessing the needs and goals of the patient and sharing ideas to address concerns together rather than working in silos. For this to work, the patient and family should remain the focus rather than the provider's individual discipline. For example, as part of an initial consultation, the palliative care physician on an interdisciplinary team conducts a psychosocial or spiritual assessment in addition to assessment of physical concerns (pain, symptoms, prognostic awareness, etc.)—with an eye for integrating other disciplines into the plan of care. Together, the team may determine that the primary concern is not physical, but rather spiritual or psychosocial. In this case, the chaplain or SW may take the lead—with an eye for the need to reintegrate the physician into the plan of care if worsening symptoms are identified (Ferrell & Paice, 2019).

At their most effective, interdisciplinary team members are able to interact dynamically such that they "make a commitment to each other to interact authentically and constructively to solve problems and to learn from one another to accomplish identified goals, purposes or outcomes" (Hamric, Spross, & Hanson, 2000, p. 318). This interaction is sometimes called role blurring. While blurring may seem to be the antithesis of role clarity, interdisciplinary teams can benefit from a bit of role blurring in which "a shared body of knowledge and skill between team members means some elements of other professionals' roles can be taken on by others if needed" (Sims, Hewitt, & Harris, 2015, p. 23), an example of which is in Box 2.8. The ability to blur effectively is, in fact, dependent on role clarity.

BOX 2.8

A PHYSICIAN REFLECTS: ROLE BLURRING AND RESPECTING BOUNDARIES

I offered to call a nursing home director once, and I thought our social worker was going to have a heart attack. She's like "that's my job!" and I said "You've taught me well! You are really busy. You have 25 other nursing homes to call, and I want to help." At first, she felt like I was mad at her—like I was saying "Oh, look. I can do your job." But I told her I knew she would have done it if she had time but she had three complicated discharges and a family meeting still today and that I'm sitting here with one patient to see and then I'm done. Working so closely together has really helped me to learn the social work aspect of things so I can help out when I need to. I also have to make sure I know my limits and remember to communicate that back to our social worker when I'm out of my depth.

To reach this ideal, each team member's core responsibilities and scope of practice must be defined and fully respected by all other members in order to avoid conflict over professional boundaries and team demoralization (Lindeke & Siekert, 2005). Bringing the best of each discipline to patient care and ensuring a consistent care experience for families requires ongoing attention to role clarity. As teams form, grow, and expand into different care settings, it is good practice to assess role clarity on a routine basis. Integrating role clarity assessments and conversations into the everyday practice of a PCT may help to guard against role confusion and personality issues (Table 2.2).

Should clarity issues arise, it is important to evaluate whether conflict is related to personality issues or role confusion. If personality conflicts are the root of the problem, the issue should be addressed at the interpersonal level rather than molding team processes around the conflict. Unaddressed conflict should not be interpreted as a lack of conflict. Contrarily, if left unaddressed, conflict can dismantle team unity and interfere with providers' abilities to perform their job duties to their fullest extent. One way to shed some light into potential areas of disagreement or friction among members may be to identify individuals' strengths (e.g., Myers Briggs, Strengths Finders, DiSC) and celebrate the diverse attributes that individuals—not just disciplines—bring to the team.

When role confusion is identified, steps should be taken to revisit the team's expectations and mission, so individuals can envision their own discipline's place

TABLE 2.2 **Results of Role Clarity and Professional Respect**

UNCLEAR COMMUNICATION ABOUT RESPONSIBILITY LEADS TO DEMORALIZATION	ROLE CLARITY AND PROFESSIONAL RESPECT ALLOWS FLEXIBILITY
Registered Nurse: This morning, I thought we agreed that I would go see a follow-up patient. I had to answer a few phone calls, and by the time I got there, our nurse practitioner had already seen the patient. When I saw her in the nurses' station, she just said, "Oh, yeah. I was right there, so I just went ahead and saw him. Don't worry about it." I know she was just trying to be helpful, but sometimes, I think I am just here to answer the phone.	**Chaplain:** Recently, one of our physicians was called into a new consult for a patient who was dying, but I was tied up in another difficult family situation. Once he realized that I was not going to be immediately available, he took the time to understand the family's spirituality. Learning that this family valued the importance of prayer, he offered to pray with them as the patient died. When the day calmed down a bit, he pulled me aside to debrief and said that he tried to incorporate the family's own spiritual language into the prayer like he has heard me do and then made a bereavement referral once the patient died. It is great to see your colleagues learning from you so they can do a good job when you are not available. You can pitch in for each other, but then go back to the work you are best at the rest of the time.

in service of the greater purpose. The following suggestions may help to facilitate this process:

1. Ensure that each discipline is practicing at the top of licensure and scope of practice by encouraging team members to serve as the "expert" in defined aspects of care.

2. Work to integrate other disciplines into the plan of care, identifying multi-dimensional needs during the initial assessment.

3. Introduce team members to patients and families using clear language to define their place on the care team even if team members will engage separately over a span of days.

4. Visit patients together when appropriate and feasible. This is an opportunity to learn from each other, build trust, and actively demonstrate roles for families.

5. Speak up if you have professional insight into issues rather than assume other team members also recognize them. Conversely, allow space for others to speak up if you are the only one contributing insight.

6. Be specific about roles in the care of particular patients, ensuring that everyone understands the plan before proceeding with care.

7. Coordinate with each other to either divide the workload equitably or carve out specific areas of accountability when roles do overlap. (Altilio & Otis-Greene, 2011; Campbell & Wood, 2012; Ferrell & Coyle, 2010).

With close teamwork over time, individual team members may become highly developed in an aspect of care traditionally handled by another discipline. It is reasonable to allow flexibility into another team member's role for temporary

---

EXHIBIT 2.1

TEAM EXERCISE FOR INTERDISCIPLINARY ROLE CLARITY

Using a scale of 0–5, with 1 being rarely and 5 being always, how often are the following statements true? Tally the responses, discuss as a team, and prioritize ways to improve.

____ I know my role on my team.

____ Others know my role on the team and respect my expertise.

____ I understand the expertise that my colleagues bring to the team.

____ I am able to practice at the top of my scope.

____ My job description actually describes what I do.

____ When I start my day, I know which patients I need to see and why.

____ I can trust my team members to flex into my role when needed.

____ My teammates trust me to flex into their roles when needed.

____ I feel comfortable sharing my opinions and perspectives.

____ Our team does a good job using the skills of all disciplines.

____ Our team intentionally takes the time to understand each other's roles.

____ We all take turns leading team meetings.

____ We all take on leadership of performance improvement projects.

____ I am a good fit for this team, and my contribution is consistently valued.

SOURCE: Adapted from Altilio, T., Dahlin, C., Remke, S., Tucker, R., & Weissman, D. (n.d.). *Strategies for maximizing health/function of palliative care teams: A resource monograph from the Center to Advance Palliative Care.* Retrieved from https://media.capc.org/filer_public/c1/87/c1879fa7-b368-401d-8e74-83f0e1ad4867/464_242_wellness_monograph_update_121.pdf

efficiency or if a patient and family prefer to work with a particular individual or discipline. However, it is also important to return to core responsibilities as soon as reasonably possible as a means to retain individual and discipline expertise. Exhibit 2.1 is an example of a role clarity exercise for PCTs. Some role overlap can be good, according to Blacker, Head, Jones, Remke, and Supiano (2016, p. 319), in that it "creates a safety net for patients and families that having 'many eyes' on a problem can assure." Only when all disciplines and individual team members feel heard can the PCT reach beyond the confines of individual disciplines when a situation calls for flexibility. This evolution from interdisciplinary to transdisciplinary teams allows for the highest-quality, comprehensive care. Further discussion about this evolution is presented in Chapter 3, Formation and Maintenance of High-Performing Palliative Care Teams.

Challenges of Role Clarity With "Borrowed" Team Members

Trust and respect are critical for high-performing teams, and it takes time and shared experiences to build teamwork. According to Rogers and Dumanovsky in CAPC's *How We Work: Trends and Insights in Hospital Palliative Care* (2017), many palliative care programs (44% in 2015), especially in smaller institutions, do not have a full, dedicated core interdisciplinary team. Of the programs that lack a full team, 70% do not have a dedicated chaplain and 54% lack a dedicated SW. Even less common is a dedicated pharmacist. The disciplines most commonly "borrowed" from the primary or other teams are SWs and chaplains. Building team norms and developing role clarity through shared experience is much more difficult, especially if these "borrowed" team members are not able to routinely participate in the team's patient care rounds. It can be helpful to include these individuals in patient care rounds (even if only in part and/or sporadically) and programmatic team meetings, as well as inviting them to participate in performance improvement projects and joining the team for informal gatherings, such as lunch (Box 2.9).

Sumser et al. (2019) note that some palliative care programs have organizational structures that, rather than aligning under a single interdisciplinary department, have team members reporting up through disciplines such as palliative care SWs under the social work department, palliative care chaplains under pastoral care, and palliative care pharmacists under pharmacy. This often results in these team members being pulled away to cover gaps in staffing, and they may find themselves stuck in competing demands, cultures, and roles.

A recent study of palliative care chaplaincy (Jeuland et al., 2017) found that chaplains who are fully dedicated to the PCT are more likely to build relationships with patients over time, care for the dying, address goals of care, and facilitate discussion with and among patients, families, and the healthcare team than

BOX 2.9

A "BORROWED" TEAM MEMBER'S PERSPECTIVE ON INCLUSION
It is a little frustrating that I can't attend palliative care rounds consistently. My department can decide to pull me away any time so the team knows to reach out if they need me for anything. With this team, you feel very comfortable. Everyone has an equal seat at the table. Whenever you start to talk, all heads turn to you, and everyone listens to what you have to say. They have asked me to work on a few projects with them, too, so I think that helped me get to know them better and they have seen that I want to contribute. When I started working with the palliative care team, I expected them to be a lot more dry and maybe kind of sad a lot of the time. Surprisingly, everybody laughs a lot. There are some inside jokes I don't always get because I'm not around as much but they really do try to keep me in the loop. Like, they ask me to come along if they are getting together after work or something.

are chaplains who are not fully integrated into a PCT. Jeuland et al. (2017) suggest that full chaplain engagement with the PCT leads to improved care of seriously ill patients.

As a matter of course, palliative care may be invited into patient care when there is some element of goal discordance, broken communication, or inadequately managed physical symptoms—after all, this is one of the essential reasons palliative care exists. According to Meier and Beresford (2007), PCT members may enter with an air of superiority, coming to rescue the patient from the primary team's failures. This "us versus them" dynamic can create a complicated working relationship with "borrowed" team members or with outside team members whose roles may blur with palliative care.

Besides affording some positive regard and a dose of humility for colleagues outside the PCT, special efforts should be made to define and integrate the roles of "borrowed" team members and with colleagues rooted in the primary care team to ensure seriously ill patients receive comprehensive, multidimensional care even when a full dedicated team is not available.

Power Differentials

According to Coyle (1997), a hierarchical tradition is deeply entrenched in the Western healthcare system. Traditionally, the physician has sole authority, and nurses and other "ancillary services" carry out orders as physicians have been positioned as the foremost experts in the delivery of patient care. This positioning leads to an implicit (and in some cases, explicit) rank order system where clinicians and caregivers from other occupations (e.g., nurses, SWs, and chaplains) may feel that their opinions and contributions matter less.

Within the biomedical model, the focus of care remains squarely on the physical domain, rendering psychosocial and spiritual disciplines almost irrelevant. The muscle memory of the biomedical model is strong, and the drive for "efficiency" can have the effect of prioritizing the physical domain at the expense of psychosocial and spiritual domains. Physicians and nurses are often presumed to be the team leaders and may automatically assume the role of facilitator for patient care meetings. Interdisciplinary team meetings that are facilitated by physicians or nurses tend to focus primarily on the physical domains of care (Parker & Peck, 2006; Wittenberg-Lyles, Cie' Gee, Parker Oliver, & Demiris, 2010).

Within the hospital setting, services provided by RNs, SWs, chaplains, and pharmacists are "bundled" into the hospital bill; they cannot directly bill for services such as physicians and APPs. As institutions look for cost-saving measures, nonbilling clinicians must constantly justify their contributions and value to the system (Blacker et al., 2016). It is often easier to lobby the executive team to hire clinicians who can directly bill for services when "worth" is demonstrated by the ability to generate revenue. Valuing "billing providers" (physicians and APPs) over "nonbilling providers" (RNs, SWs, chaplains) can also result in inequitable access to funding for professional continuing education and even acquisition of work supplies. However, this practice may shift as healthcare transitions from the traditional fee-for-service model to value-based care (Landon, 2017).

Physicians, in particular, are more likely to be invited to an institution's decision-making table, which results in increased power of resource allocation. Dahlin, Coyne, Goldberg, and Vaughan (2019) note that physicians are more likely to be contracted to work a set number of clinical hours with some protected research or administrative time than other disciplines. This tendency perpetuates the cycle of inequitable opportunities for leadership. This, and the uncomfortable reality of disparate salaries among disciplines (Table 2.3), can exacerbate power differentials within PCTs.

For PCTs to work well, reducing hierarchies is important, but changing this culture is difficult. One challenge is that the traditional gatekeepers to changing hierarchies—physicians—may either resist the change or be oblivious to its need. The study of interdisciplinary medical practice by Watson, Heatley, Gallois, and Kruske (2016) found that those with higher power (e.g. physicians) were more likely to view communication with other types of professionals (e.g., nurses and midwives) as more positive. The nurses and midwives in the study articulated less positive communication interactions with the physicians and felt that the

TABLE 2.3 **Average Salaries of Interdisciplinary Team Members**

TEAM MEMBER	AVERAGE SALARY
Physician (palliative care)	$193,559/year
Hospital pharmacist	$108,704 /year
APRN	$92,936/year
Registered nurse	$63,533/year
Medical social worker	$52,177/year
Hospital chaplain	$48,179/year

SOURCE: Data from Payscale. (2019, February 25). *Salary data and career research center*. Retrieved from https://www.payscale.com/research/US/Country=United_States/Salary

physicians viewed them as lower status partners. Since the physicians perceived the communication as mostly positive, the nurses and midwives did not believe they would be successful in changing the hierarchical culture of their organizations and win greater legitimacy for their voices.

Gibbon (1999) states, "In reality, team members do not share equality [...] This is part of the rhetoric of teamwork that is misleading at best and patronizing at worst" (p. 248). Power differentials within teams may not only be related to the dominant medical model but also may center around issues of seniority, age, gender, and race. Even though the interdisciplinary palliative care model explicitly challenges hierarchical structures, PCTs that work within traditional and societal frameworks can expect a trickle-down effect unless all team members acknowledge the tension and make conscious efforts to manage inequalities within the team (Altilio & Otis-Green, 2011).

Engaging in true interdisciplinary teamwork may rest upon the readiness of physicians to share some power. One physician, when asked why he thinks his PCT functions better than other interdisciplinary health teams at his hospital, explained,

> They [those teams] don't divide and conquer. They don't determine who's got the best skill set for the patient at that time. It's very doctor-centered still, so much so that it all starts with the doc and ends with the doc. And if a doc "needs" the nurse practitioner to go do something, then the nurse practitioner gets to do something. Their NPs are just scribes. They get a little bit of history, write it down on a piece of paper and that's it. Sometimes they [NPs] actually get to use their skill set and their brain and do something, but not very often because the docs don't use them anywhere close to their abilities. It's a real shame.

The concept of shared leadership may be especially challenging for physicians who are explicitly trained to practice and value autonomy. For this reason, according to Dahlin et al. (2019), physicians may not readily delegate clinical leadership to other disciplines or recognize the need for formal administrative leadership. Other disciplines, trained to defer to authority until specific delegation occurs, may be disinclined to accept leadership responsibility.

Those team members with less institutional power also bear responsibility in power sharing. Higgins (2011) recommends building credibility by establishing oneself or one's own discipline as the "expert" in at least one care domain. It is important to sit at the table and speak up rather than assume other disciplines are able to identify the same issues without equivalent training and expertise, especially when they may not understand another discipline's scope of practice. Though there is concern about "medicalizing" language around spirituality and human emotions, professionals rooted in the psychosocial and spiritual domains may find it useful to adopt the language of medicine. For instance, in its clinical practice guidelines, the National Comprehensive Cancer Network (NCCN) describes "diagnoses" of concerns about dying/death and the afterlife, feelings of worthlessness or being a burden, doubts about belief, grief/loss, and so forth.

Dahlin et al. (2019) offer some ideas for disrupting ingrained power structure and equalizing discourse:

- Acknowledging existing power differentials
- Formalizing interdisciplinary leadership roles
- Encouraging all disciplines to facilitate patient care or team meetings
- Having all team members address each other using first names
- Arranging for administrative time for all team members to participate in leadership or project work
- Explicitly acknowledging colleagues' expertise and role when interacting with patients, families, and other healthcare professionals

Chapter 6, Occupational Culture: Understanding the Role and Stigma of Palliative Care, expands upon the concept of working through hierarchies.

PEARLS FROM THE FIELD: TEAM TAKEAWAYS

Suffering associated with a serious illness often crosses physical, psychosocial, and spiritual domains, requiring the need to address all aspects of care. While individual healthcare providers can become skilled in these areas, expert-level care is best delivered through an interdisciplinary team of professionals with specialty training.

(continued next page)

Takeaway 1: Advocate for a full, dedicated palliative care team with representation by the core disciplines.

Ideally, PCTs will include specialty-trained physicians and nurses, pharmacists, SWs, and chaplains. While it can be challenging to convince health systems to invest in a full dedicated PCT, having all core disciplines represented allows for the development of a common mission and vision that supports comprehensive, holistic care of patients living with serious illness and their families. When a full, dedicated team is not attainable, work toward fostering collaborative relationships with individual professionals from related departments (e.g., pastoral care, social work, pharmacy) to build palliative care skills and ensure good continuity of care. Intentional efforts should be made to invite "borrowed" team members into the culture of the palliative care program by including them in patient care meetings and social gatherings whenever possible.

Takeaway 2: Clarify and respect interdisciplinary roles and expertise.

When PCT members understand their own roles and core responsibilities and respect those of their colleagues, the team is more likely to function at the highest level. In addition to the obvious benefit of close collaboration on patient care, teams that have committed to a culture of interdisciplinary respect and collegiality are able to build upon each other's skills across the care domains, develop trust, and reduce the risk of professional demoralization. Team members who feel that their expertise is understood and respected by their colleagues are more likely to feel comfortable temporarily delegating responsibilities on a busy day, trusting that their core value they bring to the team remains intact. Integrating regular, intentional communication about interdisciplinary roles into daily patient care practices allows for flexibility that can help prevent burnout. Through shared vision and explicit acknowledgment of interdisciplinary and individual expertise, PCT members can seamlessly collaborate across all aspects of care to ensure the work gets done both effectively and efficiently.

Takeaway 3: Explicitly work to break down power differentials within the team.

Without intentional efforts to acknowledge and address existing power differentials in healthcare, interdisciplinary teams are more likely to slip into traditional hierarchical roles with a heavy focus on the physical domain at the expense of the psychosocial and spiritual aspects of care. Physicians, who typically hold the most institutional power and, through their training, tend to highly value professional autonomy, may be called to "go against the grain" by sharing leadership

(continued next page)

with and advocating for other disciplines in the palliative care team. Those with less institutional power should take a seat at the table, speak up, and accept leadership opportunities. Ideas to break down power differentials include acknowledging that they exist, explicitly referring to the expertise of team members when interacting with patients and other members of the healthcare team, and sharing leadership responsibilities such as meeting facilitation and project management.

References

Abu-Ras, W. (2011). Chaplaincy and spiritual care services: The case for Muslim patients. *Topics in Integrative Health Care, 2*(2). Retrieved from http://tihcij.com/pdf/Vol2i2/chaplaincy-and-spiritual-care-services.pdf

Altilio, T., Dahlin, C., Remke, S., Tucker, R., & Weissman, D. (n.d.). *Strategies for maximizing health/function of palliative care teams: A resource monograph from the Center to Advance Palliative Care.* Retrieved from https://media.capc.org/filer_public/c1/87/c1879fa7-b368-401d-8e74-83f0e1ad4867/464_242_wellness_monograph_update_121.pdf

Altilio, T., & Otis-Green, S. (2011). *Oxford textbook of palliative social work.* New York, NY: Oxford University Press.

American Academy of Hospice and Palliative Medicine. (2019). *Workforce data and reports.* Retrieved from http://aahpm.org/career/workforce-study#HPMphysicians

American Association of Colleges of Nursing. (2004, October). *AACN position statement on the practice doctorate in nursing.* Retrieved from https://www.aacnnursing.org/Portals/42/News/Position-Statements/DNP.pdf

American Nurses Association. (2016). *Nurses' roles and responsibilities in providing care and support at the end of life.* Retrieved from https://www.nursingworld.org/~4af078/globalassets/docs/ana/ethics/endoflife-positionstatement.pdf

APRN Consensus Work Group & APRN Joint Dialogue Group. (2008, July 7). *Consensus model for APRN regulation: Licensure, accreditation, certification & education.* Retrieved from https://cdn.ymaws.com/www.nonpf.org/resource/resmgr/consensus_model/aprnconsensusmodelfinal09.pdf

Association of Professional Chaplains. (2000, September). *Code of ethics.* Retrieved from http://www.professionalchaplains.org/Files/professional_standards/professional_ethics/apc_code_of_ethics.pdf

Blacker, S., Head, B. A., Jones B. L., Remke, S. S., & Supiano, K. (2016). Advancing hospice and palliative care social work leadership in interprofessional education and practice. *Journal of Social Work in End of Life and Palliative Care, 12*(4), 316–330. doi:10.1080/15524256.2016.1247771

Campbell, T. C., & Wood, G. J. (2012). Communication and teamwork. In C. P. Storey (Ed.), *UNIPAC 5: A resource guide for hospice and palliative care professionals* (4th ed.). Glenview, IL: American Academy of Hospice and Palliative Medicine.

Coyle, N. (1997). Interdisciplinary collaboration in hospital palliative care: Chimera or goal? *Palliative Medicine, 11*(4), 265–266. doi:10.1177/026921639701100401

Dahlin, C. (2014). *Competencies for the hospice and advanced practice nurse* (2nd ed.). Pittsburgh, PA: Hospice and Palliative Nurse Association.

Dahlin, C., & Coyne, P. (2019). The palliative APRN leader. *Annals of Palliative Medicine, 8*(Suppl. 1), S30–S38. doi:10.21037/apm.2018.06.03

Dahlin, C., Coyne, P., & Ferrell, B. R. (Eds.). (2016). *Advanced practice palliative nursing.* New York, NY: Oxford University Press.

Dahlin, C., Coyne, P., Goldberg, J., & Vaughan, L. (2019). Palliative care leadership. *Journal of Palliative Care, 34*(1), 21–28. doi:10.1177/0825859718791427

Ferrell, B. R., & Coyle, N. (2008). *The nature of suffering and the goals of nursing.* New York, NY: Oxford University Press.

Ferrell, B. R., & Paice, J. A. (Eds.). (2019). *Oxford textbook of palliative nursing* (5th ed.). New York, NY: Oxford University Press.

Frieman, A., & Nowicki, K. M. (2019, January 22). *The administrative and clinical dyad: Clarifying roles & prioritizing effectively [webinar].* Center to Advance Palliative Care Webinar Series. Retrieved from https://www.capc.org/events/recorded-webinars/administrative-and-clinical-dyad-clarifying-roles-and-prioritizing-effectively-together/

Gibbon, B. (1999). An investigation of interprofessional collaboration in stroke rehabilitation team conferences. *Journal of Clinical Nursing, 8*, 246–252.

Hamric, A. B., Spross, J. A., & Hanson, C. M. (2000). *Advanced nursing practice, an integrative approach.* Philadelphia: Saunders Company.

Head, B., Peters, B., Middleton, A., Friedman, C., & Guman, N. (2019). Results of a nationwide hospice and palliative care social work job analysis. *Journal of Social Work in End of Life & Palliative Care, 15*(1), 16–33. doi:10.1080/15524256.2019.1577326

Herndon, C. M., Nee, D., Atayee, R. S., Craig, D. S., Lehn, J., Moore, P. S., … Waldfogel, J. (2016). ASHP guidelines on the pharmacist's role in palliative and hospice care. *American Journal of Health-System Pharmacy, 73*(17), 1351–1367. doi:10.2146/ajhp160244

Higgins, P. C. (2011). Guess who's coming to dinner? The emerging identity palliative social workers. In T. Altilio & S. Otis-Green (Eds.), *Oxford textbook of palliative social work* (1st ed., pp. 31–40). New York: Oxford University Press.

Institute of Medicine. (2011). *The future of nursing: Leading change, advancing health.* Washington, DC: National Academies Press.

Jeuland, J., Fitchett, G., Schulman-Green, D., & Kapo, J. (2017, May). Chaplains working in palliative care: Who they are and what they do. *Journal of Palliative Medicine, 20*(5), 502–508. doi:10.1089/jpm.2016.0308

Johnston, B., & Smith, L. (2006). Nurses' and patients' perceptions of expert palliative nursing care. *Journal of Advanced Nursing, 54*, 700–709. doi:10.1111/j.1365-2648.2006.03857.x

Landon, B. (2017). Tipping the scale. The norms hypothesis and physician behavior. *New England Journal of Medicine, 376*(9), 810–811. doi:10.1056/NEJMp1510923

Lindeke, L., & Sieckert, A. (2205). Nurse-physician workplace collaboration. *The Online Journal of Issues in Nursing, 10*(1), Manuscript 4. Retrieved from http://ojin.nursingworld.org

Meier, D. E., & Beresford, L. (2007). Consultation etiquette challenges palliative care to be on its best behavior. *Journal of Palliative Medicine, 10*(1), 7–11. doi:10.1089/jpm.2006.9997

National Consensus Project for Hospice and Palliative Care. (2018). *Clinical practice guidelines for quality palliative care* (4th ed.). Richmond, VA: National Coalition for Hospice and Palliative Care. Retrieved from https://www.nationalcoalitionhpc.org/ncp/

Otis-Green, S., Sidhu, R. K., Del Ferraro, C., & Ferrell, B. (2014). Integrating social work into palliative care for lung cancer patients and families: A multi-disciplinary approach. *Journal of Psychosocial Oncology, 32*(4), 431–446. doi:10.1080/07347332.2014.917140

Parker, O. D., & Peck, G. (2006). Inside the interdisciplinary team experiences of hospice social workers. *Journal of Social Work in End-of-Life and Palliative Care, 2*(3), 7–21. doi:10.1300/J457v02n03_03

Payscale. (2019, February 25). *Salary data and career research center.* Retrieved from https://www.payscale.com/research/US/Country=United_States/Salary

Perez, G. K. (2015). Promoting resiliency among palliative care clinicians: Stressors, coping strategies, and training needs. *Journal of Palliative Medicine, 18*(4), 332–337. doi:10 .1089/jpm.2014.0221

Pruskowski, J., Arnold, R., & Skeldar, S. J. (2017). Development of a health-system palliative care clinical pharmacist. *American Journal of Health-System Pharmacy, 74*(1), e6– e8. doi:10.2146/ajhp160055

Puchalski, C., Ferrell, B., Virani, R., Otis-Green, S., Baird, P., Chochinov, H., … Sulmasy, D. (2009). Improving the quality of spiritual care as a dimension of palliative care: The report of the consensus conference. *Journal of Palliative Medicine, 12*(10), 885–904. doi:10.1089/jpm.2009.0142

Richmond, C. (2005, July 23). Dame cicely Saunders. *BMJ, 331*(7750), 238.

Rogers, M., & Dumanovsky, T. (2017). *How we work: Trends and insights in hospital palliative care.* Retrieved from https://registry.capc.org/wp-content/uploads/2017/02/How -We-Work-Trends-and-Insights-in-Hospital-Palliative-Care-2009-2015.pdf

Sims, S., Hewitt, G., & Harris, R. (2015). Evidence of collaboration, pooling of resources, learning and role bluffing in interprofessional health care teams: A realist synthesis. *Journal of Interprofessional Care, 29*(1), 20–25. doi:10.3109/13561820.2014.939745

Stein, G. L., Cagle, J. G., & Christ, G. H. (2017). Social work involvement in advance care planning: Findings from a large survey of social workers in hospice and palliative care settings. *Journal of Palliative Medicine, 20*(3), 253–259. doi:10.1089/jpm.2016.0352

Sumser, B., Leimena, M., & Altilio, T. (2019). *Palliative care: A guide for health social workers.* New York, NY: Oxford University Press.

Watson, B. M., Heatley, M. L., Gallois, C., & Kruske, S. (2016). The importance of effective communication in interprofessional practice: Perspectives of maternity clinicians. *Health Communication, 31*(4), 400–407. doi:10.1080/10410236.2014.960992

Wittenberg-Lyles, E. M., Cie' Gee, G., Parker Oliver, D., & Demiris, G. (2009). What patients and families don't hear: Backstage communication in hospice interdisciplinary team meetings. *Journal of Housing for the Elderly, 23*, 92–105. doi:10.1080/02763890802665007

CHAPTER 3

FORMATION AND MAINTENANCE OF HIGH-PERFORMING PALLIATIVE CARE TEAMS

Introduction

Given the difficulties of getting any team, let alone a healthcare team, to work together well, it may seem easier to just go forward with an individual discipline or multidisciplinary model for palliative care teams (PCTs). However, research and theory agree that the severity of the health conditions addressed by palliative care providers and the complexity of the medical, social, psychological, and spiritual concerns of palliative care patients and families demand a team approach to care (Connor, 1998). Moreover, the best care of patients and families results from an interdisciplinary model (Ledford, Canzona, Cafferty, & Kalish, 2016), and PCTs are better situated to navigate the complex work environments of hospitals. So, while it may seem hard, the best answer to this problem is to learn how to build and maintain interdisciplinary teams.

Negative Palliative Care Experience

Social Worker Perspective: It's so frustrating. The nurses act like I have nothing to add when a patient is suffering because I'm "just a social worker." ... there was a patient who was complaining of abdominal pain. I knew that the pain medicine she was taking causes constipation, and I noticed from the chart that she hadn't had a bowel movement for 5 days. Now, I'm not a nurse, but it seemed reasonable to consider that might be the problem. The nurse shut me down and told me that wasn't my job.

Positive Palliative Care Experience

APRN Perspective: People are so open to learning. One of the things I've seen on this team is a great desire to be taught by fellow team members. On the really bad

A podcast to accompany this chapter is available with online access of this title. Please see the instructions on the first page of the book for details on how to access and go to Chapter 3.

teams I've worked with, it was "I know everything, and you don't." This one is "I really don't know everything, and I'm sure there are a million things, so tell me what I don't know. I really do want to learn that. Let's figure this out together."

Teamwork in Palliative Care

As awareness of palliative care needs grows and hospitals become increasingly willing to commit staff resources to meet this need, so grows the understanding of the breadth and depth of physical, emotional, and spiritual stressors faced by seriously ill patients and their families. Considering the scope of the challenges and needs that patients and families face during times of serious illness, it becomes clear that the expertise of several disciplines is the best way to provide patient-centered care. PCTs are often the answer to this call. However, just as palliative care is a different way of doing healthcare, the building of PCTs is also a different venture than most of the team-building experiences that healthcare professionals have had in training and professional settings. While there is clear evidence that multidisciplinary and interdisciplinary teams contribute to patient and professional satisfaction and improved patient outcomes (e.g., Epstein, 2014; Lemieux-Charles & McGuire, 2006), this is not how the medical education system is oriented (Schottenfeld et al., 2016). Additionally, PCTs interact with other multidisciplinary hospital departments such as cardiology and oncology, which can create a double-edged sword and introduce additional challenges into an already complex medical system (see Box 3.1).

BOX 3.1

A NURSE REFLECTS: WORKING WITHIN A COMPLEX SYSTEM

As a palliative care nurse, I have to be aware of how and to whom I communicate. If I go to oncology and say "I don't know what you guys are smoking, but this plan you think you have for this patient is terrible." That is never going to fly. But if I go to the nurse and find out what's going on there, go to the aides and find out what's going on there, talk to the social worker, talk to the family, talk to the patient, get the entire lay of the land, and then find the oncology nurse practitioner, and say "Here is the way the landscape really looks. I know you think it looks like X on the surface, but it really is Y." When they say "Oh, that's going to be a problem," I say "I'm just bringing you this information so that everyone has the whole picture." Then what you'll see over the next 2 days are nurse practitioners saying to the oncologist "FYI, palliative care uncovered this big mess. It's going to make our plan not work." Initially, the oncologists really got their hackles up that palliative was in there messing up their plan. They are starting to understand that letting us help them get the whole picture results in a plan that works for everybody.

One reason that multidisciplinary groups experience challenges in connecting and working together as a whole is because we tend to be drawn to those who are similar to us. This can result in some group identity issues that can be blinding in the face of multidisciplinary problem-solving. Tajfel and Turner's (1986) social identity theory (SIT) shows us that once individuals identify with a particular group—such as with other nurses or physicians—they will favor the perspectives of that group (their ingroup) and downplay, reject, or ignore the perspectives of other professionals (their outgroups). You may recognize this basic human tendency when you reflect on the last time you joined a new team, when you had someone new join your team, or as you work to strengthen and maintain existing team relationships. As palliative care is multidisciplinary by nature, those working within the specialty will likely experience both task and emotional challenges as they work to start and maintain teams within the larger hospital/healthcare system setting (outgroup). The double-edged sword appears as PCTs find themselves strategizing to best work with other teams in the hospital (outgroups) yet simultaneously find themselves shut out of conversations that could help their patients (Watson, Heatley, Gallois, & Kruske, 2016). This blocking occurs because the outgroup (e.g., oncology) views working with the PCT as less important than the patient care plan already established or, at worse, as failure in medicine on the part of the referring group.

If other departments do not seek or accept the insights and opinions of PCTs, it is difficult for the PCT to feel it has done its best on the part of the patient. Moreover, if that PCT does not have a strong team foundation to begin with, organizational challenges, such as a lack of communication with other departments, can erode the confidence of the PCT and create increasing frustration among team members with other staff and with the larger organization in which they work.

▶ Moving From I to We: Beyond Multidisciplinary Teams

Healthcare is evolving from a traditional focus on single-provider care to embracing team-based care. In addition to blending multiple provider perspectives, research shows that teams are less prone to mistakes than are individuals (Baker, Day, & Salas, 2006). Box 3.2 offers an example.

▶ An accompanying video, Everybody Overlaps in an Interdisciplinary Team, presenting a physician's perspective from Dr. Elizabeth Grady, may be accessed at connect.springerpub.com/content/book/978-0-8261-5806-2/ch03.

BOX 3.2

A SOCIAL WORKER REFLECTS: IT'S IMPORTANT TO KNOW WHAT YOU DON'T KNOW

In my last job, we had an executive director who was a very successful businesswoman, and her second career was as a director of this nonprofit for cancer care where I was a social worker. She had personal experience with cancer, and so she felt that there was no problem kind of being a clinician when she didn't have the background or the license. And it was really hard. First of all, she was my boss, but there wasn't a sense of respect for my role, so it was a difficult conversation to have with her about what she didn't know and what she shouldn't say to patients and their families and what promises she should not make. She did not take it well, but she doesn't have a license in my field. My current team understands how to be transdisciplinary and so we can talk more easily about how to know what we don't know. That makes a difference for our team and our patients and families. We are fortunate to have a team that can talk like this.

This increase in patient safety stems from the following (Johnson, 2019):

- Team members' ability to consult one another
- Collaboration to consider potential consequences or benefits of a course of treatment
- Building consensus or agreement among team members
- Streamlining the complexity of the healthcare system
- Decreasing the need for patients to see a multitude of specialists
- Increased provider communication about cases via formal and informal communication (e.g., rounds, patient visits, encrypted messaging, hallway conversations)

Figure 3.1 shows the evolution of healthcare from an early focus on one provider to the aspirational transdisciplinary team. In their seminal work tracing the transition from individual expertise to collective approaches to patient care, Choi and Pak (2006) suggested that while multidisciplinary, interdisciplinary, and transdisciplinary approaches illustrate a continuum of varying degrees of integration, each approach has a unique word to describe its focus:

1. **Multidisciplinary = Additive**
   What does this look like in the healthcare setting? A patient is individually assessed by a variety of specialists (e.g., psychologists, nutrition, cardiology) while under the care of a lead provider (such as a bariatric surgeon).

2. **Interdisciplinary = Integrative**
    What does this look like in the healthcare setting? A variety of providers, such as a counselor, primary care physician, and psychiatrist, discuss their individual assessments and collaborate to develop a comprehensive care plan for the patient.

3. **Transdisciplinary = Holistic**
    What does this look like in the healthcare setting? While providers' disciplinary identities (e.g., nurse, physician, social worker) serve as their core expertise, they seek to enhance patient care by teaching and learning from other team members. Therefore, a palliative care physician may see that a nurse can perform roles that he or she was trained for but can also learn to take on new responsibilities such as helping to mitigate family dynamic issues (a skill learned from working closely with social workers).

Interdisciplinary teams are now considered the gold standard of patient-centered care and a hallmark of palliative care. Due to the complexity of caring for seriously ill patients and their families, an evolution to transdisciplinary teams is aspirational for the field of palliative care. It is important to consider how teams form and what team leaders and members can do to establish and maintain a high-performing interdisciplinary program.

Team Formation and Maintenance

Once a healthcare system or healthcare facility decides to start a PCT, they set off down the road of team formation. All teams, regardless of industry or purpose, undergo similar stages through which they grow. The standard means for understanding these stages is Tuckman's (1965) five-stage model (Figure 3.2). It is important to note that this model was designed to explain short-term groups or task forces as well as permanent teams. Therefore, the fifth stage of the model, adjourning, is not relevant for most PCTs. It is also important to remember that stage models are great for understanding what might happen at particular stages, but their linear appearance can be misleading. Human interaction rarely follows a linear path, and thus, the interacting lines and arrows on this model remind teams that returning to an earlier stage—for instance, when there is a change in team membership or a refocusing of function—is a normal part of the process. Returning to earlier stages is not only normal, it is often a healthy way for teams to address conflict, integrate new members, regroup, and grow as a group.

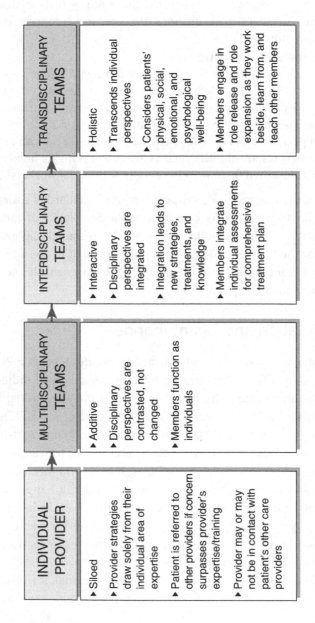

INDIVIDUAL PROVIDER

▶ Siloed
▶ Provider strategies draw solely from their individual area of expertise
▶ Patient is referred to other providers if concern surpasses provider's expertise/training
▶ Provider may or may not be in contact with patient's other care providers

MULTIDISCIPLINARY TEAMS

▶ Additive
▶ Disciplinary perspectives are contrasted, not changed
▶ Members function as individuals

INTERDISCIPLINARY TEAMS

▶ Interactive
▶ Disciplinary perspectives are integrated
▶ Integration leads to new strategies, treatments, and knowledge
▶ Members integrate individual assessments for comprehensive treatment plan

TRANSDISCIPLINARY TEAMS

▶ Holistic
▶ Transcends individual perspectives
▶ Considers patients' physical, social, emotional, and psychological well-being
▶ Members engage in role release and role expansion as they work beside, learn from, and teach other members

FIGURE 3.1 Evolution to transdisciplinary healthcare teams.

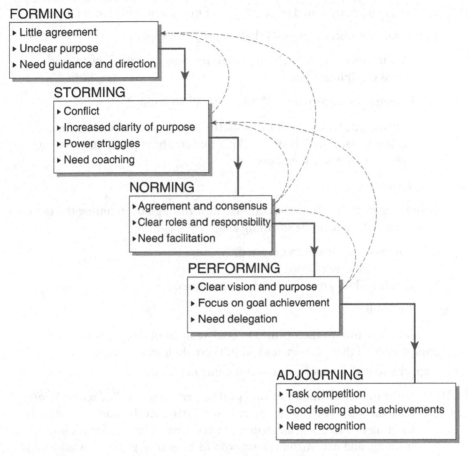

FIGURE 3.2 Tuckman's (1965) stage model for groups.

SOURCE: Data from Tuckman, B. W. (1965). Developmental sequence in small groups. *Psychological Bulletin*, 63, 384–399. doi:10.1037/h0022100

Stage 1: Forming

Team members begin interacting.

Ground rules are identified.

- ■ Stage characterized by both energy and uncertainty.
- ■ Usually leader-driven.

Stage 2: Storming

Disagreements of varying levels of severity occur.

May encounter strong emotional responses.

Conflict causes include a mix of issues concerning ideas, personal identity, and team identity.

Issues may be exacerbated by two types of uncertainty in team members.

- Predictive uncertainty = "What is going to happen?"

  May include questions about how to become a group, how to work across disciplinary lines.

- Explanatory uncertainty = "Why is this happening?"

  May include issues about the sometimes intense nature of the interdisciplinary team, anxiety over talking openly about group processes, or events that trouble members.

Stage 3: Norming

Group begins to function as a cohesive unit through overcoming the issues that occurred while in the storming stage.

- Interpersonal structures created.
- Open exchange of information.
- Emotional support of fellow team members.

Stage 4: Performing

As they work toward their common goal, team confidence grows in the competence of their teammates and in their abilities as a team.

Capacity to problem-solve and adapt continues to grow.

- Some models include a second part of performing called *outperforming* (Manges, Scott-Cawiezell, & Ward, 2016). At the stage, the team is meeting or exceeding all goals and may send members for additional training, add new members, or expand or update goals. New additions in strategies and personnel can build a "re-energized group" (p. 27). As with any stage, adding new elements makes it likely that the team will return to the earlier stages of storming and norming although the length of time in those stages may be shorter.

Stage 5: Adjourning

While not true for all teams, some teams end. For short-term problem-solving groups and special task forces, once the team has met its goal, it will likely disband. For work teams that have long-standing goals such as customer service or the care of patients and families at the end of life, this stage will likely only be realized if the organization decides to disband, merge, or otherwise change the fundamental nature of an ongoing group. When adjourning is the next step for a group, this stage may be resisted by members who enjoy the relationships and synergy of the team even though they recognize that the purpose of the team is completed.

Next, the team development stages are applied specifically to PCTs.

Stage 1: Forming a New PCT

Given the rapid growth of PCTs in various hospital settings, the question of when to start a PCT could be at one of several stages on the continuum of PCT preparedness (Figure 3.3).

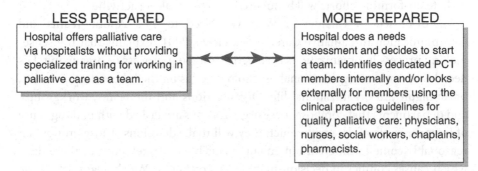

FIGURE 3.3 Organizational preparedness for palliative care team (PCT) creation.

If a team is starting from scratch, the best practice is to try and establish who the team is at the beginning through conscious questioning and careful discernment (Box 3.3). For example, through observation and interviews with a high-performing PCT at St. Martha's Hospital (pseudonym), Imes and Hester (2014, 2015) describe team formation that included a negotiated period of preparation when they were on payroll but not yet taking referrals. During that time, the team met frequently, got to know one another, and asked themselves the questions in Exhibit 3.1. These are *who*, *what*, and *how* questions and address both internal team communication (ingroup) and communication with others in the hospital (outgroups). The process of talking their way into these answers for a still-emerging structure is a form of creating and understanding for future use of the ideas, otherwise known as cognitive mapping. Cognitive mapping is useful even in beginning team stages, as it establishes frames, or common ways of understanding, onto which further team development will be built.

BOX 3.3

A FOUNDING PCT MEMBER REFLECTS: PREPARING TO MAKE A TEAM

It was a blank slate. We really started with "How are we going to do this? What does this look like?" About a year ago, I was cleaning out my computer files, and I found this document from our planning time. It's funny to look back on it because it seems like our processes today are what we've always done with little changes, but that came from that preparation time of really intentionally talking about how we were going to do this.

How do we know who we are? Social identity theorists Tajfel and Turner (1986) note that a primary purpose in group formation is the identification of ingroups and outgroups. Many of the questions posed in the forming process concern discovering team boundaries as well as linkages to groups or disciplines. The forming process for teams setting out to be a new kind of team means that much of the early team-forming efforts will be focused on sensemaking activities.

As discussed in Chapter 1, Why We Need to Talk About Teams and Communication in Palliative Care, Weick (1995, 2001) explains that the sensemaking process in organizations is an active, ongoing process of organizing. His decades of work in organizational psychology focus on the inherent *equivocality*, or ambiguity, in organizational life. Organizations and the teams, workgroups, and departments that compose these organizations are tasked with making sense of large amounts of data with which they will make decisions. Those groups can reasonably come to different but equally plausible interpretations of these data, which causes conflict in decision-making. According to Weick, teams that have *requisite variety* have the best chance to engage in sensemaking that is meaningful and effective. For Weick, *requisite variety* means that those involved in sensemaking have a greater breadth and complexity of experience and knowledge than is required to make sense of the problem in a useful way. All that breadth is used to match the inherent ambiguity in decision-making with a collective mind that has sufficient ability to understand and solve problems (Weick, 2005). If we could measure complexity by volume, Weick is saying that a 16 oz. problem is best tackled by a group with at least 18 oz. or more of problem-solving capacity.

This notion of requisite variety is the very reason that healthcare teams function as a means of effective patient care. Lemieux-Charles and McGuire (2006) found that "the type and diversity of clinical expertise involved in team decision-making largely accounts for improvements in patient care and organizational effectiveness" (p. 263). Their review of the literature found that teams that were more integrated, or interdisciplinary rather than multidisciplinary, made better use of their greater breadth of knowledge and experience. To combine the theories of SIT and sensemaking, teams that use their requisite variety to make efficient sense of the data may form a social identity as a thriving, high-performing team.

Looking again to the exemplar team at St. Martha's Hospital, the newly forming PCT worked intentionally to consider the question "Who are we?" from the very beginning of their forming process. Starting out with the recommended core members of a palliative care team (physician, APRN, social worker, and chaplain), they had the requisite variety needed to serve the seriously ill patients and families in this hospital through the comprehensive palliative care model.

However, having all the right people does not mean that the team will become high performing. The St. Martha's team asked the questions in Exhibit 3.1 as a means of sensemaking, which also served to form their social identity in the hospital. This process can take some time as team members navigate one another's personalities and initial expectations. However, teams that do not invest the time in such processes may find it difficult to ever answer the question "Who are we?" with more than "A loosely connected group of professionals."

The questions in Exhibit 3.1 cover a variety of domains. If a team is already formed and functioning, consideration of the questions in this exhibit remains important and can help teams figure out avenues to improve team communication and processes.

EXHIBIT 3.1

FORMING STAGE QUESTIONS

Identity Questions	Communication Channel Questions

Who are we?
• What are our roles?
  • What do you do?
  • What do I do?
  • What do we bring to this team?
• Should there be overlap in our roles?
• What happens to workflow when there is overlap?
	What will we use to communicate?
	• What kinds of technology do we use when we are not talking face-to-face?
	  • Email? Texting? Encrypted messaging?
	• Which channel is appropriate for which content?
	• Are there any subjects or times we should avoid using technology to communicate and talk face-to-face or make a phone call rather than type?

Ingroup Communication Questions	**Outgroup Communication Questions**

How do we talk with one another?
• Do we address one another by first names?
• Are we going to talk with one another throughout the day or save most work talk for meetings when everyone is there?
• How are we going to meet?
  • How often?
  • When?
• What kinds of meetings should there be?
  • How do we know if our meetings are working?
	How do we talk with others in our organization?
	• How will we talk about our PCT as a group to other groups in the hospital?
	• What do we call ourselves?
	• Is how we interact with outside groups different if we are interacting just as ourselves or as representatives of our PCT?
	• How will we get other departments to refer patients to us?
	  • Is there a process we set now?
	  • How will we know if the referral process is working?

The St. Martha's PCT also utilized a work styles inventory early on in their forming stage and discovered some major differences in work style preferences. As they worked through their questions (Exhibit 3.1) of identity and communication, they would ask each other about the interaction of their style preferences and continually affirm the importance of the variety of their work styles to how well their team was working together. Affirming responses, even of those who had varied style preferences, helped to establish or reaffirm the interpersonal relationships among members. While teams often think of themselves as a group that has tasks to perform, the questions in Exhibit 3.1 indicate that team communication has both task and relational components. Tasks might include how to document patient care in a team-based model or whom to contact if the team pharmacist is unavailable for a consult. Relational components include how team members will handle conflict and even something as seemingly simple as how team members will address one another.

For PCTs, the forming stage is a great time to address power differentials on the team that are based on disciplines. Historically, physicians have been afforded higher power status in healthcare settings. On PCTs, physicians are important members; however, the collaborative team-based model calls for all members to find relatively equal seats at the table. In organizational cultures where some members of the team are routinely called by their first name, all members should be called by their first name when speaking with each other. In the forming stage, teams are advised to discuss the necessary efforts to "leave their egos at the door," so to speak (Box 3.4).

BOX 3.4

A SOCIAL WORKER REFLECTS: IS IT REALISTIC TO BELIEVE WE CAN LEAVE EGO AT THE DOOR?

We try to leave ego at the door as much as we humanly can, but I think a strong ego is good to have in this setting because you do get beat down so much by so many people outside of the team. So, I appreciate a strong, healthy ego. It's just people knowing their boundaries—kind of back to the scope of practice. So I love that our nurses are rock stars in pain management and how they deal with symptoms, and I want them to be rock stars as nurses—at the same time, they know they're not social work rock stars. Once again, it's about the boundaries and scope of practice about what everyone does. It goes back to the mutual respect for what we all do.

Stage 2: Storming

The storming stage is a necessary part of team formation, yet members often find it unsettling. After the idea generation processes that occur in the forming stage, the storming stage refines ideas and begins to make choices. Those choices will involve resource use as well as processes that may be outside of some group members' comfort zones. The disagreement that generally comes with those choices at this stage can be particularly hard for indirect communicators or those who identify as shy or conflict averse. Some groups who made it through to the performing stage note that the storming stage was where they nearly stopped the process and disbanded (Manges, Scott-Cawiezell, & Ward, 2016). However, if teams wish to achieve their objectives, it is important that they overcome the resistance and tension in the storming phase and focus instead on productive conflict management skills. It is often most effective if conflict management is facilitated by the team leadership and not left only to the most vocal members of the group.

When productive conflict occurs in the storming stage, groups work their way through choices and discover where their perspectives align or diverge from the team. The process may be uncomfortable for some due to the direct nature of handling dissent that is often used on teams for decision-making. However, with intentional management of the discussion and healthy communication guidelines in place (established in the forming phase), the process should not harm individual identities or the team's cohesiveness. Learning to differentiate among debate, discussion, and dialogue and determining when each is best applied is one way that teams can build their constructive conflict management skills (Exhibit 3.2).

If the team devolves into destructive conflict, a focus on "winning" for individual points of view may encourage communicative actions designed to hurt members' feelings and even their credibility. Such tactics may be employed as a disincentive to productive dissent. While the destructive tactic may "win" the point, it often results in a "loss" to the team's health.

The tendency to employ destructive communication styles can be increased when one group believes its legitimacy is questioned by another group. PCTs are caught in a perceptual bind—they understand their role of assisting patients and families dealing with serious illness, but the professionals with whom they interact to fulfill their role may demean the existence of their specialty. This negative interaction with outgroups may threaten the social identity of the newly forming PCT. As team members feel stressed by these interactions with outgroups, their communication may become less competent and amplify uncertainty and

EXHIBIT 3.2

DIFFERENTIATING AMONG DEBATE, DISCUSSION, AND DIALOGUE

	DEBATE	DISCUSSION	DIALOGUE
COMMUNICATION	Two sides oppose each other for the purpose of proving the other wrong Positions asserted forcefully Creates closed-minded attitudes	Exchange of information, opinions, expertise Little attention paid to power or status Helps formation of an abstract notion of community	Two or more sides work together toward achieving a common understanding Understanding based on appreciating differences and personal experience
SELF-ORIENTATION	Defends own position as the best solution Excludes other solutions Avoids revealing one's assumptions	Primary goal is to clarify and understand the issue Assumes all positions are grounded in a stable reality Orientation toward being right	One submits one's best thinking, knowing that other people's reactions will help improve it rather than destroy it Members reveal assumptions and personal values
OTHER ORIENTATION	Listens in order to find flaws and weaknesses in the other positions Aim is to critique and defeat	Listens in order to insert one's own perspective Little regard for the participation of others	Listens in order to understand through finding meaning and points of connection Searches for strengths in other positions Oriented toward modifying one's perspective
EMOTIONS	Unconcerned with feelings and emotions of the other team members Does not consider how debate will affect the relationship with the others	Emotional responses may be present but are not welcomed Strong focus on content over relationship	Emotions are welcomed as they help to deepen the understanding of the personal and group relationship issues
GOAL	Win	Encourage multiple perspectives	Find common ground

SOURCE: Compiled and adapted by Nadga et al. (2009) based on "Differentiating Dialogue from Discussion," a handout developed by Kardia and Sevig (1997) for the Program on Intergroup Relations, Conflict and Community (IGRC), University of Michigan; and "Comparing Dialogue and Debate," a paper prepared by S. Berman, based on discussions of the Dialogue Group of the Boston Chapter for Educators for Social Responsibility (ESR). Other members included L. Burt, D Mayo-Smith, L. Stowell, and G. Thompson.

feelings of anxiety already present in the storming stage. This threat to group identity and the professional pride of the PCT increases emotional investment in the conflict. The challenge of legitimacy is not unusual for PCT providers, as explored by Omilion-Hodges and Swords (2017):

- "I learned early on that if I don't clearly articulate what I do and why it's important, I'm treated like a leper."
- "I wish that others understood what I really do. In addition to monitoring a patient and tending to their physical needs and helping them to manage their pain, I get to know them. I ask them questions. I don't set a broken arm and send the patient away—I become part of the family and treat them all."
- "It [disrespectful treatment] comes to a head when they've just released someone to my care—especially if it's a patient they've been with a while. I know that they [the physicians] are hurting, but telling me 'it's time to pretend you're useful' is not the optimal way to ask me to care for a patient" (p. 1278).

While this threat to legitimacy comes from outside the group, it can still affect group formation and group identity. In some ways, it may bond the group closer and help them through the storming stage. However, anything external to the group that increases the anxiety and uncertainty of group members may also exacerbate the conflicts they have within the group.

The Coordinated Management of Meaning Model (Cronen, Pearce, & Snavely, 1979) focuses on how people create their communication environments, and, according to their model, "we get what we make." One of the ways that we get problematic communication is through participating in repetitive, deteriorating communication patterns. This theory describes a serpentine model for these patterns to show how triggers and reactions lead people down a path that is unhelpful but hard to change (Pearce, 2008). PCTs may more easily recognize these patterns with outgroups (Figure 3.4A), but they can also occur within the PCTs (Figure 3.4B). In a serpentine conversation, each person's turn is an opportunity to take the conversation in a different direction. In these two cases, each person's turn is used to attack or defend. If just one participant chooses a more productive response, the outcome of the conversation may be different. In the case of repetitive patterns of deteriorating communication, that one choice to make this conversation different may result in a more productive starting point the next time these providers interact.

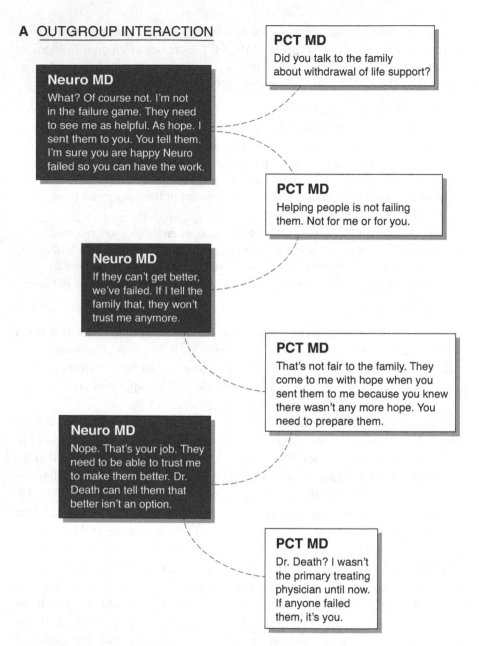

A OUTGROUP INTERACTION

> **PCT MD**
> Did you talk to the family about withdrawal of life support?

> **Neuro MD**
> What? Of course not. I'm not in the failure game. They need to see me as helpful. As hope. I sent them to you. You tell them. I'm sure you are happy Neuro failed so you can have the work.

> **PCT MD**
> Helping people is not failing them. Not for me or for you.

> **Neuro MD**
> If they can't get better, we've failed. If I tell the family that, they won't trust me anymore.

> **PCT MD**
> That's not fair to the family. They come to me with hope when you sent them to me because you knew there wasn't any more hope. You need to prepare them.

> **Neuro MD**
> Nope. That's your job. They need to be able to trust me to make them better. Dr. Death can tell them that better isn't an option.

> **PCT MD**
> Dr. Death? I wasn't the primary treating physician until now. If anyone failed them, it's you.

FIGURE 3.4A Serpentine conversations showing deterioration.

In both of these examples, the focus is on winning the ego game. If asked, everyone involved would say that patient care is the most important part of what they do. Yet both of these conversations leave the patient care conversation quickly

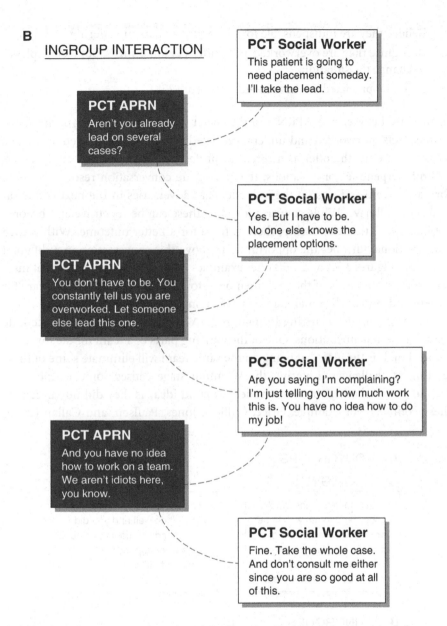

FIGURE 3.4B Serpentine Conversations Showing Deterioration (*continued*)

and become embroiled in a battle of wills where winning the point becomes more important than caring for the patient. For Figure 3.4A, the problem is exacerbated by the neurologist's challenge to the PCT physician's legitimacy as a healthcare provider. For Figure 3.4B, the underlying martyr's syndrome as described by Weissman (2011) is a significant factor. Weismann proposes that team members experiencing the following may be "palliative care martyrs" (p. 1278) who:

- Believe they are indispensable for managing all patient suffering
- Recognize they are overworked and under personal stress, but feel helpless to change the situation
- Feel unappreciated by those in authority (p. 1278).

In the case between the APRN and the social worker in Figure 3.4B, the social worker feels overworked and underappreciated. When help is offered, the social worker perceives the offer as a threat to professional identity and competence. In both serpentine conversations, the end of the conversation resolves nothing for patient care and sets up the individuals as adversaries in the next conversation they will have. While conversations like these can be repetitive and become debilitating to the relationship, there is hope for a better outcome. Within each conversational turn lies the opportunity to move this conversation in a different direction. Figures 3.5A and 3.5B offer examples of alternative responses that meet the professional needs of the PCT member—to provide the best possible care for patient and family while maintaining professional dignity with colleagues.

Much of what is occurring in Figures 3.4A and 3.4B stems from inaccurate perceptions and attributions. One of the enticing parts of a team model for many professionals is the idea that being on the same team will eliminate some of these legitimacy challenges. Entering the storming stage causes some members to second-guess whether the team model is a good idea, as they did not anticipate these conflicts. For example, Grice, Galliois, Jones, Paulsen, and Callan (2006)

A   OUTGROUPS

ORIGINAL

> That's not fair to the family. They come to me with hope when you sent them to me because you knew there wasn't any more hope. You need to prepare them.

TRY THIS

> It's hard when a patient doesn't do well and you did everything you could to help. Let's work together to talk with the family.

B   INGROUPS

ORIGINAL

> You don't have to be. You constantly tell us you are overworked. Let someone else lead this one.

TRY THIS

> You do such a great job for our patients and I've learned so much from you. Let me help you.

FIGURE 3.5 Alternative ways to communicate.

studied a large psychiatric hospital undergoing significant restructuring. One of the keys to the success of this transition was the extent to which team members were willing to share information with one another. Their findings on team communication point out the complexity of identity on work teams and some of the stumbling blocks no one saw coming such as inaccurate perceptions of the behaviors of fellow team members. They identified the following membership types: double ingroup, partial ingroup, and double outgroup. To see these identities in action, consider an APRN on a PCT of 14 people (Figure 3.6).

Grice et al. (2006) hypothesized that team members "would report sharing more information with double ingroup members than with partial ingroup members" (p. 335). However, their study found no significant difference in actual information sharing among team members. What they did find was a perception by team members that they received more information from double ingroup members than partial ingroup members when, in fact, the evidence did not support that perception. This means that this APRN (Figure 3.6) might feel more trust in the competency of her double ingroup colleagues because she thinks she is getting more information from them than from team members such as physicians or social workers. These perceptions may be particularly damaging in the early stages of team development. If left unchecked, this type of inaccurate perception is just one of many factors that can eat away at a team's foundations and lead to Weissman's (2015) observation of PCTs moving away from what can be their greatest strength—strong interdisciplinary bonds.

Adept communication practices can assist teams in observing these problems as they are and avoid the pitfalls of inaccurate perceptions and attributions. Martin and Nakayama (2018) offer seven suggestions to deal with interpersonal conflict:

1. Stay centered. Do not polarize.
2. Maintain contact.
3. Recognize the existence of different styles.
4. Identify your preferred style.
5. Creatively expand your style repertoire.
6. Recognize the importance of conflict context.
7. Be willing to forgive. (p. 461)

One PCT physician discussed how mindful planning for communication and conflict does not mean it always goes the way he wants. He says, "When I'm on palliative service I think, as I'm driving in, 'I wonder who I'll meet today and what I'll need to respond to today?' And I just hope that I'm able to respond appropriately. So, you have that going into it, intentionally looking for it and thinking about patients and communication challenges. It just makes it interesting but also hard, you know? You learn a lot from people." However, there will be cases where

DOUBLE INGROUP
MEMBERS

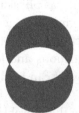

When employees are members on
both a work team and
occupational group

SAME TEAM, SAME DISCIPLINE:

Common educational background
means easier communication
shortcuts

Empathy is easy to find and express
when someone does the same job
as you do

Problems can occur if the similarity in
background is conflated with doing
everything exactly the same as
another person would

Example: Other APRNs on her PCT

PARTIAL INGROUP
MEMBERS

When employees are
ingroup members for the work team
OR occupational group but
outgroup members on the other

SAME TEAM, DIFFERENT DISCIPLINE:

Common PCT communication
shortcuts and ingroup references

May cause conflict through
purposeful or inadvertent
characterization of other
disciplines as less important to
patient care

SAME DISCIPLINE, DIFFERENT TEAM:

Educational background short
cuts for meaning making

Fundamental misunderstandings of
palliative care may mean conflict
through statements that make
palliative care seem unimportant

Examples: Physicians, social workers,
chaplains, and pharmacists on her PCT
OR
Other APRNs at her hospital

DOUBLE OUTGROUP
MEMBERS

When employees are members of
neither the work team nor the
same occupation

DIFFERENT TEAMS, DIFFERENT
DISCIPLINES:

Long-standing disciplinary power
differentials may be difficult to
address or overcome

Misunderstandings about
palliative care may lead to
professional jealousy over use
of resources (hires, promotional
materials) for PCTs

Example: Healthcare providers/
employees at the hospital who are not
on her PCT and are not APRNs (i.e.,
cardiologist or oncology social worker)

FIGURE 3.6 Ingroup, partial ingroup, and outgroup membership for an APRN on a PCT with 14
other team members.

conflict is particularly hard to resolve. When it seems dialogue is at an impasse, Back, Arnold, and Tulsky (2010) suggest reflecting on three questions:

1. How important is this to the other person's core beliefs/values?
2. How important is this to my own core beliefs/values?
3. How flexible can I be without compromising an important value of my own? (p. 104)

Box 3.5 offers an example of examining core beliefs and values to resolve conflict through consensus.

Stage 3: Norming—Identifying as a Team

As the team begins to achieve equilibrium due to the choices it makes through the storming process, the norming stage may begin. Some team characteristics of PCTs that thrive may emerge in the norming stage. These characteristics include enacting the team as a group of bonded believers and interdependent interdisciplinarians, contributing to cohesive communication in the group, and communicating the value of the team and of team members to one another as well as to other individuals and groups.

BOX 3.5

THE VALUE AND VALUES INHERENT IN LUNCH

PCT members had a disagreement about whether it was appropriate to accept lunches from hospice organizations who were hoping to generate more referrals. Most team members did not feel strongly about this issue, but one nurse who had previously worked for a hospice felt that providing the team with lunches was the only way some of the smaller hospices had to differentiate their services. She also liked having lunches provided, noting that it seemed to improve the team's morale. One of the physicians believed strongly that it was unethical to accept gifts from outside organizations, a stand she'd taken early in her career. Several side discussions occurred over months with increasing degrees of conflict. At an impasse, the PCT held a formal meeting to come to consensus. Through discussion, the nurse realized that the practice of accepting lunches was a core belief for the physician, whereas this issue was not as important to her own values. The team came to consensus that they would not accept lunches and, addressing the nurse's concerns about access, the nurse agreed to become the team's point person for hospice organizations. PCT members also started bringing in more snacks to share to address the team morale issue.

Bonded Believers and Interdependent Interdisciplinarians

In high-performing, low-turnover PCTs, every member of the PCT is a believer in the mission of the team. The PCT model appeals to them because it moves beyond the silo model through which most were educated. Within their teams, members often articulate the necessity of their work, and they may express despair for hospitals that do not have a PCT model. One APRN said, "I know a palliative care nurse at another hospital in town. She's it. No team. I can't imagine how she gets through her day. The worst part is that there is just no way those patients and families are getting the same level of care in that hospital." Members of a high-performing group often have backgrounds of participation in PCTs that failed due to underfunding or understaffing, or they come from hospital settings that did not have PCTs at all. For these members, the perception of a strong foundation of the team's purpose is affirmed through regular communication among team members about the importance of their work and their gratefulness for their team experience. Although moving from the silo model of medicine to the interdisciplinary or transdisciplinary model can be a dramatic and sometimes stressful change, the benefits of interdependence manifest in their work with patients and work with their team.

Teams often bond through processing experiences together. Designated PCTs spend a lot of time together. They may eat lunch together, walk to meetings together, and get together socially outside of work hours. In highly bonded teams, much of their workday talk is not just reporting to one another but also processing work experiences together (Box 3.6).

BOX 3.6

PROCESSING COMMUNICATION

Dietra, an APRN, enters the office first thing in the morning and immediately starts to talk with Taylor, an RN, about an interaction with a non-PCT physician from the day before: "... And he yelled at me! The patient does not like reality, and I was bringing up something that was going to make that doc talk to the family. And he yelled at me!"

Taylor commiserates with Dietra about the inappropriateness of that reaction from a hospital colleague, and they look at the text exchange between Dietra and the physician following the face-to-face interaction. Taylor notes that Dietra really disarmed the doctor's annoyance with the tone of the text, and they both agree that this colleague gets a little more latitude than others might because he really is a nice person. When rounds begin a few minutes later, this doctor and patient are first on the list, and Taylor says

"And Dietra got yelled at . . ." while Dietra ruefully laughs. The rest of the team asks for the story and agrees that it is yet another hard case, and this doctor usually reacts more appropriately. They continue processing the case, catching up on the chart, and getting input from all the team members who interact with this patient before deciding the next steps.

Additionally, whether it is talk about work, conversation to process work events, or just chatting about their everyday lives, members and teams that communicate frequently and freely tend to feel more supported and experience higher levels of trust with their peers (Omilion-Hodges & Ackerman, 2018). This may stem from the fact that over time, the continued communication leads to peer and team cohesion.

Cohesive Communication

Cohesive communication occurs when group members use similar words or phrases when talking with their team or about their team. This type of communication increases as the team spends more time together. While team members might purposefully choose words or phrases to describe themselves in the forming process (see Exhibit 3.1), emergence of higher levels of cohesive communication occurs organically as members pick up phrases from one another simply through the repetition made possible by spending a lot of time together. One type of cohesive communication, word matching (Gonzales, Hancock, & Pennebaker, 2010), or parallel storytelling is a good indication that a team has cohesive communication. Norrick (2000) found that retelling known stories indicates that group members feel involved and their parallel language use shows careful attention to how and why stories are told in the group. This storytelling serves to ratify their group membership and make sense of what happens in their group. This agreement on the meaning of situations allows teams to feel greater satisfaction in their team experiences, as they believe they understand others and are understood by others. PCTs with high volume and frequency of communication may exhibit spontaneous parallel storytelling between team members and when reflecting on their experiences with others outside the team. This is to say that in reminiscing or making a point to one another or individuals outside of the team, multiple group members may tell the same story from their own perspective. This story would have a high degree of fidelity among each version even though it was told from a different individual's perspective.

For example, during interviews with St. Martha's high-performing team, all 15 members were asked about the formation of the team 5 years before—their origin story. The eight members who were part of the original team told very similar stories, including key decisions, concerns, and celebratory moments. Interestingly, the seven members who joined the team in the years since also tell the story while acknowledging that they were not present to see it happen. This parallel storytelling shows that the team uses this origin story as an orientation for new members and that it is also a key component of the story they tell about their identity (Imes & Hester, 2014, 2015). Elements of the story that influence this particular team include early decisions to try to avoid typical hierarchies on the team, belief in the importance of the work they do and how working with this team makes it possible, and feelings of gratitude that they have the opportunity to be on such a team. Narrative processing of this type was common for this PCT, so much so that they come back to the same stories and find the reliving of those moments to be bonding for the storyteller and listener.

Communicating Value

Team members show they value their colleagues professionally through both explicit and implicit statements. Expressions of

- "That's a good catch!"
- "Would you mind taking a crack at this case?"
- "Your skills with this patient are better than mine for this situation."

are a means of validating the worth of a colleague. When statements of this kind are made with regularity and received by group members without pause, this indicates that the team finds professional compliments normal. For St. Martha's PCT, all team members mentioned that they felt valued. When asked how they knew that they are valued by the team, most answered "Because they tell me all the time that I am."

Another way that team members may express that they are feeling valued is by comparing a current situation that they like with a past situation where they did not feel valued. For example, St. Martha's PCT was making a conscious effort to follow the best practice guidelines of ensuring that every patient had a spiritual assessment. The team chaplains mentioned that the spirituality portion can be sidelined with some teams. However, during rounds with this team, if there is no spiritual assessment noted in the chart, the chaplain at the meeting is always asked to perform one. While this request added to their considerable workloads, it also meant that their work is valued because the team cares if the assessments are not done.

While it is recommended that team leaders encourage and model frequent praise of members, the importance of communicating value within teams becomes clear when PCTs run into difficulties. If every member is seen as vital, what happens when someone is gone? As a PCT gains the trust and respect of its hospital and colleagues, the patient census will continue to grow. Thus, missing a member from the team for any reason means more work for everyone. While members are often trained in role flexing to accommodate patient needs and team resources, functioning understaffed for long periods of time can lead to burnout and/or compassion fatigue (Back, Rushton, Kaszniak, & Halifax, 2015). Beyond the workload, it throws off the balance of the team dynamics. Some team members note that this is an annoying price to pay for being so valued that you can never be gone. However, in the same breath, members usually say it with a smile and acknowledge the reality that team members will get sick and need to go on vacation from time to time. In the case of vacation time, absences are preplanned and the team may be able to prepare. However, when unexpected absences occur on the team, the whole team feels the significant stress (Box 3.7). Illness may be the most common unexpected absence, but in high-stress positions such as palliative care, last-minute decisions by one member may have considerable effects on the team.

Communication Point People

One of the tasks of norming on interdisciplinary teams means figuring out your communication hubs. Without adept internal and external communication, even a team of kind, smart people who love palliative care work will not thrive as a team; they probably will not even survive as a team. Many PCTs have a formalized coordinator role (often an RN) who serves as a communication hub for patient care.

BOX 3.7

A CHAPLAIN REFLECTS: DEALING WITH UNEXPECTED ABSENCE WHILE COMMUNICATING VALUE

I just got so overwhelmed. I took a few days off and didn't tell anyone on the team ahead of time or try to get another chaplain to cover me. When I got back, my colleagues sat me down, and do you know what the first question was? The very first thing they said was "Did you think we wouldn't miss you?"

The chaplain received this opening to what was ultimately a reprimand situation as an affirmation of her importance to the team. The PCT workload was difficult to balance but even as she was reprimanded, the team chose an expression of value to explain what her absence meant to the team.

This team member simplifies communication with the PCT by serving as a single point of contact and a conduit of information between the team and others to ensure coordination of care. Like all team positions, it is important to find a good fit for the coordinator role, as this position is vital to effective team functioning.

In high-performing teams, other types of communication hubs may emerge as well. Often functioning at an informal level, one highly trusted person may serve the role of coordinating interpersonal team member communication.

> *Who will talk to people about how they talk to people? I will. If one of the social workers is having a conflict with a physician, just tell me where you need me to go. I will advocate for this team by making sure they talk to one another. Within the team, I just remind people that we are in this together. This work is too important, so let's just figure this out, talk—we're adults.—Catie, APRN*

Some teams may identify another primary communicator to work with outgroups. For example, a team physician with connections in administration may serve as the PCT's advocate at the administrator level. In general, teams that are conscientious about the choice and fit of their communication hubs begin to model the type of communication seen in successful intentional communities.

Stage 4: Performing

Once norming is achieved, teams may feel they have accomplished their team construction and they are done working on the team. At this stage, the team may want to know—are we a good team? Remember the criteria delineating minimally performing teams from high-performing teams from Chapter 1, Why We Need to Talk about Teams and Communication in Palliative Care.

Once teams reach the performing stage, the fourth part of Tuckman's model, they may be somewhere on the continuum between the minimally and high-performing criteria (see Table 1.1 in Chapter 1, Why We Need to Talk About Teams and Communication in Palliative Care). While it is true the team exists, the real test is if the team maintains its practices. This stage is more than continuing to replicate the practices from the norming stage—the performing team is still a verb; it must continually re-create itself in order to succeed.

The performing stage usually goes well as long as the team continues to practice intentional communication. One model for considering intentional communication in high-performing teams is the concept of intentional communities. Even though many think only of intentional communities as the explosion of the utopian commune communities of the 1960s and 1970s (Holden & Schrock, 2007), such arrangements have existed for thousands of years (Love Brown, 2002) and can be used as a model to better understand the maintenance of intentional communication in high-performing PCTs.

Traditionally, five criteria are used to determine the designation of an intentional community:

- Use of consensus in decision-making
- Shared/negotiated value system
- Shared residence
- Team-based goals
- Constructive marginalization (Kamau, 2002; Love Brown, 2002; Mulder, Costanza, & Erickson, 2006; Olsen, Jason, Davidson, & Ferrari, 2009; Sanguinetti, 2012)

While PCTs do not co-reside in the way usually described by intentional communities, high-performing transdisciplinary teams share many qualities with effective intentional communities (Table 3.1).

As a model, intentional community brings what is most important to high-performing PCTs—a continuing focus on intentionality. After all of the work to create a team through the forming, storming, and norming processes, this team must be maintained. Maintenance requires consistent attention and follow-through. Teams that do not commit to the maintenance of what they have built and continue to engage in discussions and actions that will lead them to where they want to be in the future will not remain high-performing. Thus, a focus on the intentionality of the communication that builds and maintains high-performing teams is a useful model.

Achievement of Team-Based Goals

Team-based goals, or super-ordinate goals, are those that an individual cannot achieve on his or her own. This criterion for intentional communication is often the impetus for starting PCTs in the first place and is required to meet the goal of high-quality care for seriously ill patients and their families. This core purpose of PCTs can be helpful in communication with stakeholders outside of the PCT, too. For hospitals that offer palliative care through hospitalists and without a designated PCT, the reaction to the implementation of a PCT may not be uniformly positive. Hospitalists could resist the suggestions from PCTs because they might not know how a PCT could enhance patient care. Dr. Stacie Pinderhughes (2015; Center to Advance Palliative Care [CAPC] palliative interview on April 26, 2015) reports using questions like "Is it hard for you to talk to patients about roles?" or "Do you have fears about prescribing opioids or benzodiazepines for symptoms?" and then she responds with "We can help with that!" Given all of the work to achieve the previous stages of team formation, a PCT might not think of itself as new even though the hospital in which

TABLE 3.1 **Intentional Community at Work**

WHAT IT LOOKS LIKE	WHAT IT SOUNDS LIKE ON PALLIATIVE CARE TEAMS
Shared work spaces	Referring to dedicated palliative care team space as "home"
	"It's exhausting out there. I'm glad to get back to the office with my people."
Team goals	"I'm glad you were on today. Taking on this situation by myself would have been a nightmare."
Shared values	"Mr. Jones died yesterday. He had a good death."
Consensus	"We've talked about this a lot—we really need to make a decision. It sounds like everyone is leaning toward this solution. Is that what we are saying?"
Constructive marginalization	"Thank goodness for this team. No one else understands me!"
	"Did you hear how they talked about palliative care at that meeting? I was insulted, but also … we know they are never going to get it, so it is a good thing we get it!"
	"Someone just asked me how it feels to be part of the 'failure' team on the hospital. I think he sincerely wanted to know. I pretended I didn't hear him and came back here as quick as I could."

it is embedded still thinks of the PCT as new. In this case, even though the PCT is at the performing stage, hospital colleagues may not understand their purpose and may undervalue the possibilities of working with the PCT. Without referrals from hospital colleagues, PCTs cannot achieve their objectives. Dr. Pinderhughes's response is "Let the hospitalists know that the formation of a PCT does not question their competence, but rather it can help to make their work life easier through the specialized knowledge of such teams." Her framing is a subtle and positive reminder to colleagues about team-based goals—we cannot achieve them on our own and that is particularly true in healthcare (see Box 3.8).

Shared/Negotiated Value System

The value systems for honoring the importance of palliative care in the lives of patients and families are at the core of why people decide to work in palliative care. They reinforce this value communicatively through reiterations of ideas and questions that center on "What does the patient need?" Problem-solving that starts with a question that focuses on the patient helps keep teams oriented to the reason most wanted to work in palliative care in the first place—to best meet the needs of patients.

BOX 3.8

AN APRN REFLECTS: ALLEVIATING DISTRESS OF NONPALLIATIVE CARE STAFF
During rounds, we talked a lot about a really difficult case in the ICU, which helped us process our feelings. We were concerned that the ICU nurses and physicians were struggling, too, and they wouldn't necessarily have an outlet for their distress. Our physician assigned to the case planned to reach out to the ICU physician to offer support, but we also assigned one of our APRNs to check in with the bedside nurses every day, and we planned a formal debriefing led by our chaplain.

For interdisciplinary teams to function well, the power hierarchies they either overcame or learned to live with as they transitioned from the storming phase to the norming phase must continue to be reiterated. Not all power hierarchies will be resolved to the complete satisfaction of everyone on the team. For example, while the majority of team members address each other by their first names, one may insist that his or her formal title is used. However, any compromises that allow the team to move forward together must be either continually upheld or even challenged for more progressive views on power-sharing (Box 3.9). If teams agree on a particular means of demonstrating respect for their colleagues and find themselves quickly backsliding into the pre-agreement ways, the team will find themselves back in the storming stage (see Table 3.2).

Another place to identify a team's shared/negotiated value system is in its expression and uses of humor. Healthcare work has long been associated with "dark" or "gallows" humor. One provider pointed out that the use of this type of humor on teams is a sign of trust. They have spent enough time together to negotiate what is appropriate for humor for their ingroup. Another team talked about an ongoing happy hour discussion they have that they find entertaining:

> We were at happy hour and making a joke about if we get arrested for disturbing the peace, what do we do? So we talked about it. If we get arrested and leave a nurse behind, she's going to make sure they [the jail] let you use the bathroom and ask "Are they feeding you?" The chaplain is going to say "We're praying for you. Have hope!" The physician is going to show that authority thing. The pharmacist is going to ask "Do you need something to calm you down?" But the social worker is the one who's going to spring you. So if we all get arrested, we need to leave the social worker behind because none of these other disciplines know what that's all about. —Callie, APRN

BOX 3.9

DEMONSTRATING RESPECT: AN EXAMPLE OF THE POTENTIAL TO RETURN TO THE STORMING STAGE

One PCT agreed during the forming stage to always use first names rather than titles when addressing one another. Core group members reported the gentle teasing of one physician on the team who routinely utilized the professional title of "Dr." when referring to team colleagues with doctoral degrees in professional settings outside of the PCT. Though he laughed it off when this practice was mentioned in his interview, it was apparent that the titles remained important to him. It was notable that within the group, he was willing to abide by the group norms, using first names for forms of address. At the same time, team members generally utilized his professional title when referring to him outside the group.

The team finds this funny because, while somewhat reductive for each position, each role is portrayed positively. It affirms each discipline's worth to the team while constructing a scenario they find hysterical—the arrest of their entire PCT.

Constructive Marginalization

Constructive marginalization means existing in the margins and is another criterion for intentional communities that PCTs fulfill. PCTs often function as outgroups in hospitals due to their unique place in the health system—caring without necessarily curing—and their unique structures as interdisciplinary groups. However, while marginalization may be viewed as a negative in other contexts, for some PCTs, it is freeing. PCTs, like other intentional communities, can thrive in their marginalization as they are less constrained by the organization; as one physician pointed out, "We get to just do our own thing and care for people. Just care for people. I think other specialties are jealous of us for that."

Watson et al. (2016) remind us that individuals are more likely to discriminate against outgroups. Even when PCTs are enjoying their marginality in some respects, they still may find themselves targeted by other outgroup members. Factors that increase discrimination against outgroups include:

- Perceived threat from competition for scarce resources
- Uncertainty about how to implement policy in critical situations
- Status/power differences among staff.

Numerous examples in this and in other chapters show that low level panic about resource use in hospitals seems to be normative as well as conflicts that are really based on status differences. Recognizing why dissent exists may help team leaders to differentiate the articulation of different ideas and points of view for the purpose of gaining a full picture of the situation from true obstruction for the purpose of being obstructive.

Use of Consensus

Consensus building can be an important element of cohesive teams. Making decisions by consensus means that everyone on the team agrees with the solution or plan. If a team is voting and following the majority vote, that is not consensus. Building consensus can be a time-intensive process. At the beginning of consensus building, team members are learning about what is important to others as well as themselves. Early in the process, this can be a struggle. Team members may name one thing, "patient care," as a reason for their objection to an idea when really it is their concern that their discipline is not being respected. As they begin to accurately identify what underlies team members' perceptions and preferences, the process speeds up because the conversation is focused on working those perceptions and preferences into alignment. If teams have been conscious of negotiating their shared value system, consensus building will come easier.

One of the benefits of taking the time to participate in consensus building is that teams tend to be more invested in the solutions they helped to create. A team with high levels of team member ownership that can articulate both its shared value system and why all the team members are necessary to achieve the superordinate goals would be a dream team. Once this level of functioning is achieved, however, team members must continue to invest efforts in mindful communication with others and great problem-solving behaviors every day to stay at this level. In many ways, the high-performing interdisciplinary team is like a garden. The gardener may spend years cultivating the space, protecting the plants, and innovating the processes, but if the gardener lets the space go for just one season without working on it, the garden will quickly revert to all of the problems the gardener spent years overcoming. The gardener can get the space back to the optimal growing and production levels that once existed, but it will take more resources. Working to maintain the high-performing team does require attention and continued resources but not as many as trying to rebuild the team after neglect.

Teams should be wary of "fake consensus." In true consensus, everyone agrees to a common solution, one that would not necessarily be considered ideal to any one individual but is acceptable to the team as a whole. In fake consensus, the dissenters do not share their dissent so it appears that everyone agrees when, in fact, they do not. This misperception will become apparent quickly, as team members either do not do what the team thought they agreed on or when they appear unwilling to commit the time and effort necessary to perform the agreed-upon functions well. This inevitably leads to conflict within the team. From the outset, fostering a culture that encourages dissent and demands compromise may seem burdensome and time-consuming. This may be true initially, but significant time can be saved through team buy-in and, ultimately, through a better solution.

Better decision-making comes to teams who dissent as a part of their process because they are better at discovering and discussing hidden profiles (Schulz-Hardt, Brodbeck, Mojzisch, Kerschreiter, & Frey, 2006). Hidden profiles occur when only part of the information is shared among group members prior to decision-making while one or more elements are unshared. The member(s) who possess the unshared elements are not necessarily hiding them; rather, it does not occur to them to share the information. Teams that allow for and encourage dissent are more likely to discover the hidden profiles and therefore have more information with which to make their decisions. Schulz-Hardt et al. found that "because dissent groups exchanged more information about the best alternative and repeated it more often, they were more likely to solve the hidden profile" (p. 1090). In other words, dissent assists teams in not moving past a point where more information was needed to make the best possible decision.

Dissent also helps to avoid groupthink (Janis, 1982). While this book and others focus on the importance of cohesion for strong teams, a team may experience groupthink when a desire for group harmony overrides the ability of members to express dissent (Table 3.2). Dissent is a part of productive conflict because it brings critical thinking into team decision-making. Additionally, the solutions proposed processes mired in groupthink may be less likely to happen anyway. If team members were agreeing because it is nice to agree, they may be less invested in enacting the solution. If they "go along to get along," they often count on the person who had the idea to carry out the solution, and that is the antithesis of the purpose of PCTs, as their strength lies in their interdisciplinarity. Teams who engage in productive conflict and arrive at a decision by consensus have a higher likelihood of championing their ideas and leading their implementation. Teams who learn to identify when groupthink is happening can avoid the pitfall while still maintaining group cohesion as long as productive dissent is encouraged as a normalized process for the team. For more about groupthink and the culture of team decision-making, look to Chapter 6, Occupational Culture: Understanding the Role and Stigma of Palliative Care.

When a team is forming, the efficacy of the processes and whether or not the team will like or even abide by these processes are unknown. Also, in the moment of forming, it may seem like communication and decision-making are clear, but the proof is in how the team experiences the structure and processes. An indication that clear communication led a process can be found in the storytelling of the team members. On St. Martha's PCT, all team members tell their PCT's origin story in a similar way. Those who are founding members have more details and are able to share information about how they were feeling but may not have shared with the group. However, the basic details of the story, including critical junctures in their journey, are virtually the same among the storytelling of different members. Even members who joined in later years recall the story as they heard it told to them. This parallel storytelling indicates that much of the identity

TABLE 3.2 What It Looks Like When We Prioritize Harmony Versus Conflict in Group Interactions

WHEN WE _____	WE OFTEN SEE _____
Prioritize group harmony first	First solution as good enough
	Less ownership
	Less follow through
	Possible apathy
	Seemingly relaxed nonverbal participation—there's less stress if you don't have any ownership and won't be held responsible for the outcome
Have productive conflict	Verbal and nonverbal engagement at varying levels based on individual comfort with dissent
	Possible hesitation that grows into higher group energy
	Multiple solutions offered
	Pros and cons of solutions weighed
	Champions of certain solutions often become owners and drivers of the solution if it is selected
Have destructive conflict	Few solutions, if any
	Personal attacks rather than problem-focused solutions
	Focus on "bringing down the opposition" or "winning your point" regardless of the expense to the other team members
	Tense and even frightened nonverbal engagement
	Conversations/meetings end to avoid more difficulty regardless of whether a solution is suggested or selected

work that the team did in the forming stages continues throughout the years. They tell their origin story to one another either as an orientation story for new members, as a reference story to consider how things have changed or if a change needs to be made, and as a bonding story as they laugh and commiserate about the work it takes to make and maintain a team.

PEARLS FROM THE FIELD

Palliative care is a complex world and requires teams adept at processing that complexity. This intense work environment is best done by interdisciplinary teams; building and maintaining those teams is an intentional process. Teams that focus on intentional communication, planning, and self-reflection throughout this process are most likely to not only become high-performing teams for patient and family care, but to be teams that survive and thrive.

Takeaway 1: Process matters

Communication is often portrayed as easy because most everyone can talk and teams are obvious because groups exist. Yet most all team members feel stress that is directly tied to the success of communication among team members and between the team and outgroup members. Growing from a new group to a performing group is not simple. Awareness of the ways in which groups form and what skills to focus on in each stage can help your team avoid some of the pitfalls of group formation. Great groups are the result of intentional communication and attention to group processes. While the process can be a lot of work, it is work worth doing for a high-performing team.

Takeaway 2: Conflict does not have to be your favorite activity, but it will happen so make it productive

All teams have conflict. If there is no conflict, then it is probable that your team is not authentically communicating with one another and it is likely that frustrations exist that are not voiced to the group. Productive conflict is good for your team. One of the purposes of teams consisting of multiple disciplines is to combine the expertise and perspectives into one solution. Everyone will not always start out in agreement, but if you can make it a productive discussion with contributions from all voices that are respected by all members, your team has a good chance at making a high-quality decision and improving team relationships.

(continued next page)

Takeaway 3: Even if you have built a fabulous high-performing team, you will lose it without attentive maintenance.

In the media and in movies in particular, a lot of attention is paid to the forming and breaking of relationships. While that may be good fodder for the viewing public, the everyday communication within relationships and teams is what makes or breaks the relationships in the long run. Teams are full of humans, and human relationships do not have, to quote an old infomercial, a "set it and forget it" function. The most mentally and emotionally taxing stages for teams are usually the forming and storming stages. However, throughout a team's life, returns to earlier stages are normal and returning to storming happens more frequently when teams stop maintaining and attending to their intentional communication practices. Like most high-quality outcomes, there is no easy path, and it is a path you must continue to walk together to find success as a team. Team communication does get easier, and as long as the team remains intentional about their processes and communication, it can remain easier. Neglect those processes and take relationships for granted and you may have quite a bit of repair work to do. Teams can return to high-performing once again, but it is easier to maintain and make slight corrections than it is to find yourselves in need of a major course correction. High-performing teams are the dream for many; if you have one, it is worth the effort to maintain it.

References

Back, A., Arnold, R., & Tulsky, J. (2010). *Mastering communication with seriously ill patients: Balancing honesty with empathy and hope.* New York: Cambridge Press.

Back, A. L., Rushton, C. H., Kaszniak, A. W., & Halifax, J. S. (2015). "Why are we doing this?": Clinician helplessness in the face of suffering. *Journal of Palliative Medicine, 18*(1), 26–30. doi:10.1089/jpm.2014.0115

Baker, D. P., Day, R., & Salas, E. (2006). Teamwork as an essential component of high--reliability organizations. *Health Services Research, 41*(4 Pt 2), 1576–1598. doi:10.1111/j .1475-6773.2006.00566.x

Choi, B. C., & Pak, A. W. (2006). Multidisciplinarity, interdisciplinarity and transdisciplinarity in health research, services, education and policy: 1. Definitions, objectives, and evidence of effectiveness. *Clinical and Investigative Medicine, 29*(6), 351–364.

Connor, S. R. (1998). *Hospice: Practice, pitfalls, and promise.* Washington, DC: Taylor and Francis.

Cronen, V., Pearce, W. B., & Snavely, L. (1979). A theory of rule-structure and types of episodes and a study of perceived enmeshment in undesired repetitive patterns (URPs). In D. Nimmo (Ed.), *Communication Yearbook 3* (pp. 225–240). New Brunswick, NJ: Transaction Books.

Epstein, N. E. (2014). Multidisciplinary in-hospital teams improve patient outcomes: A review. *Surgical Neurology International, 5*(Suppl. 7), S295–S303. doi:10.4103/2152 -7806.139612

Gonzales, A. L., Hancock, J. T., & Pennebaker, J. W. (2010). Language style matching as a predictor of Social Dynamics in Small Groups. *Communication Research, 37*(1), 3–19. doi:10.1177/0093650209351468

Grice, T. A., Gallois, C., Jones, E., Paulsen, N., & Callan, V. J. (2006). "We do it, but they don't": Multiple categorizations and work team communication. *Journal of Applied Communication Research, 34*(4), 331–348. doi:10.1080/00909880600908591

Imes, R. S., & Hester, J. (2014). *Loving group work: Is this is Holy Grail of group communication? Investigating a transdisciplinary palliative care team.* Paper presented at the National Communication Association Annual Convention, Chicago, IL.

Imes, R. S., & Hester, J. (2015). *Unintended intentional community at work: Applying a new lens to guide the formation and maintenance of transdisciplinary teams.* Paper presented at the National Communication Association Annual Convention, Las Vegas, NV.

Holden, D., & Schrock, D. (2007). "Get therapy and work on it": Managing dissent in an Intentional Community. *Symbolic Interaction, 30*(2), 175–198. doi:10.1525/si.2007.30 .2.175

Janis, I. L. (1982). *Groupthink: Psychological studies of policy decisions and fiascoes.* Boston: Houghton Mifflin.

Johnson, J. D. (2019). Framing communication in health care action teams. *International Journal of Healthcare Management, 12*(1), 68–74. doi:10.1080/20479700.2017.1398386

Kamau, L. J. (2002). Liminality, communitas, charisma, and community. In S. Love Brown's (Ed.), *Intentional communication: An anthropological perspective* (pp. 17–35). Albany, NY: State University of New York Press.

Ledford, C. J. W., Canzona, M. R., Cafferty, L. A., & Kalish, V. B. (2016). Negotiating the equivocality of palliative care: A ground theory of team communicative processes in inpatient medicine. *Health Communication, 31*(5), 536–543. doi:10.1080/10410236 .2014.974134

Lemieux-Charles, L., & McGuire, W. L. (2006). What do we know about health care team effectiveness: A review of the literature. *Medical Care Research and Review, 63*(3), 263–300. doi:10.1177/1077558706287003

Love Brown, S. (Ed.). (2002). Introduction. In *Intentional communication: An anthropological perspective.* Albany, NY: State University of New York Press.

Manges, K., Scott-Cawiezell, J., & Ward, M. M. (2016). Maximizing team performance: The critical role of the nurse leader. *Nursing Forum, 52*(1), 21–29. doi:10.1111/nuf.12161

Martin, J. N., & Nakayama, T. K. (2018). *Intercultural communication in contexts* (7th ed.). New York: McGraw-Hill Education.

Mulder, K., Costanza, R., & Erickson, J. (2006). The contribution of built, human, social and natural capital to quality of life in intentional and unintentional communities. *Ecological Economics, 59*, 13–23. doi:10.1016/j.ecolecon.2005.09.021

Nagda, B. A., Gurin, P., Sorensen, N., Gurin-Sands, C., & Osuna, S. M. (2009). From separate corners to dialogue and action. *Race and Social Problems, 1*, 45. doi:10.1007/s12552-009-9002-6

Norrick, N. (2000). *Conversational narrative: Storytelling in everyday talk.* Amsterdam, The Netherlands: John Benjamins Publishing.

Olsen, B., Jason, L. A., Davidson, M., & Ferrari, J. R. (2009). Increases in tolerance within naturalistic, intentional communities: A randomized, longitudinal examination. *American Journal Community Psychology, 44*, 188–195. doi:10.1007/s10464-009-9275-3

Omilion-Hodges, L. M., & Ackerman, C. D. (2018). From the technical know-how to the free flow of ideas: Exploring the effects of leader, peer, and team communication on employee creativity. *Communication Quarterly, 66*(1), 38–57. doi:10.1080/01463373 .2017.1325385

Omilion-Hodges, L. M., & Swords, N. M. (2017). The grim reaper, hounds of hell, and Dr. Death: The role of storytelling for palliative care in competing medical meaning systems. *Health Communication, 32*(10) doi:10.1080/10410236.2016.1219928

Pearce, W. B. (2008). *Making social worlds: A communication perspective.* Malden, MA: Blackwell.

Pinderhughes, S. (2015, April 26). *Palliative care: The needs assessment* [Video file]. Retrieved from https://www.youtube.com/watch?v=9I8O18dVQbc

Sanguinetti, A. (2012). The design of intentional communities: A recycled perspective on sustainable neighborhoods. *Behavior and Social Issues, 21*, 5–25. doi:10.5210/bsi.v20i0 .3873

Schottenfeld, L., Petersen, D., Peikes, D., Ricciardi, R., Burak, H., McNellis, R., & Genevro, J. (2016). *Creating patient-centered team-based primary care.* Rockville: Agency for Healthcare Research and Quality.

Schulz-Hardt, S., Brodbeck, F. C., Mojzisch, A., Kerschreiter, R., & Frey, D. (2006). Group decision making in hidden profile situations: Dissent as a facilitation for decision quality. *Journal of Personality and Social Psychology, 91*(6), 1080–1093. doi:10.1037/0022 -3514.91.6.1080

Tajfel, H., & Turner, J. C. (1986). The social identity theory of intergroup behavior. In S. Worchel & W. G. Austin (Eds.), *Psychology of intergroup relations* (pp. 7–24). Chicago: Hall Publishers.

Tuckman, B. W. (1965). Developmental sequence in small groups. *Psychological Bulletin, 63*, 384–399. doi:10.1037/h0022100

Watson, B. M., Heatley, M. L., Gallois, C., & Kruske, S. (2016). The importance of effective communication in interprofessional practice: Perspectives of maternity clinicians. *Health Communication, 31*(4), 400–407. doi:10.1080/10410236.2014.9609222

Weick, K. (1995). *Sensemaking in organizations.* Thousand Oaks, CA: Sage.

Weick, K. (2001). *Making sense of the organization.* Oxford: Blackwell Publishers.

Weick, K. (2005). Managing the unexpected: Complexity as distributed sensemaking. In R. R. McDaniel & D. J. Dreibe (Eds.), *Uncertain and surprise in complex systems: Question on working with the unexpected* (pp. 51–78). Berlin: Springer-Verlag.

Weissman, D. E. (2011). Martyrs in palliative care. *Journal of Palliative Medicine, 14*(12), 1278–1279. doi:10.1089/jpm.2011.0293

Weissman, D. E. (2015). Improving care during a time of crisis: The evolving role of specialty palliative care teams. *Journal of Palliative Medicine, 18*(3), 204–207. doi:10.1089/ jpm.2015.1014

CHAPTER 4

LEADING PALLIATIVE CARE TEAMS

Introduction

The importance of great team leadership cannot be overstated. While a team may survive a poor leader, they are unlikely to thrive and may experience high turnover and high stress levels. Both of these undesirable outcomes can negatively impact the care of seriously ill patients and their families. Leadership also impacts the very ability of teams to work together well. Palliative care is delivered in the team-based format to utilize the knowledge, skills, and talent of several disciplines as a cohesive unit. Teams with poor leadership are unlikely to get beyond the multidisciplinary stage to the more effective and efficient interdisciplinary or even transdisciplinary stage. Great team leaders model intentional communication, understand how to mediate conflict, work to nurture individual team member development, and are attentive to the development of the team as a whole. Great team leadership makes a big difference in the complex world of palliative care.

Negative Palliative Care Experience

Nurse Practitioner Perspective: *It's hard to figure out the reporting structure for the team. We have the medical director and that's who the hospital says is the lead, but mostly in name only because every discipline still reports up through their own structure even though we work together on this team. So I report up through a nursing director who really doesn't communicate at all with our medical director, and she is from a totally different service line, which is confusing. Our chaplains report up through pastoral services, and our social workers report to the social work department—they can get pulled from our team without much notice if that department has someone out. It feels like people are always pulled in so many directions. We have trouble getting all these leaders to see the whole picture for our team. Even figuring out how to order things like paper can be hard.*

A podcast to accompany this chapter is available with online access of this title. Please see the instructions on the first page of the book for details on how to access and go to Chapter 4.

Positive Palliative Care Experience

Physician Perspective: *We've always had informal leaders on our team—those who take on most of the strategy, organizing our process. Our APRN is the one who initially took on things like making sure we had a time and place for our team meetings, setting the agenda, and keeping us on track. We all work together to figure out how we want to do things like documentation, but it was understood that she would put legs on the plan by partnering with IT to make it work. As the medical director, I'm asked to present our outcomes to administration and argue the case for more resources. It goes against the system's grain, but I always ask her to present the work.*

Best Practices of Team Leaders

Teams are indispensable to the delivery of palliative care. Part and parcel with high-performing palliative care teams are committed ethical team leaders (Cutler, Morecroft, Carey, & Kennedy, 2019; Dahlin, Coyne, Goldberg, & Vaughan, 2019). What characteristics make up a strong palliative care team (PCT) leader?

- A strong communicator who can influence members to work toward a common goal
- A focus on shared leadership and collective accountability
- Ability to articulate and appreciate individual team roles and member expertise
- A patient-centered focus
- Establishing and fostering a clear team purpose and commitment to the interdisciplinary team
- Encouraging all members to participate while balancing member participation (managing dominant members, engaging more tentative members)

Palliative care leaders may be formal (titled) or informal. Formal leaders are often administrative leaders (e.g., managers) who are explicitly tasked to manage personnel, budgets, operational processes, and business planning or are clinical leaders (e.g., medical director) who direct staff training and competencies, clinical processes, and referral relationships. See Chapter 2, Who Are the Players? Exploring the Types of Palliative Care Providers, for more information about administrative versus clinical leadership roles. Informal leaders may be any PCT member (e.g., APRN) who, though not titled, takes on strategy and systemization of team processes or serves as a respected mentor. Informal leaders may or may not be recognized for their work or be acknowledged with the authority that is proportionate to their lived role within a hierarchical administrative structure (Dahlin et al., 2019). If not, formal leaders should take care to highlight and recognize the work of informal leaders, ideally inviting them to a "seat at the table."

BOX 4.1

POPULAR DEFINITIONS OF LEADERSHIP

"Leadership and learning are indispensable to each other." —John F. Kennedy

"Leadership is about making others better as a result of your presence, and making sure that impact lasts in your absence." —Sheryl Sandberg

"Successful leadership is leading with the heart, not just the head. [Leaders] possess qualities like empathy, compassion and courage." —Bill George

"I start with the premise that the function of leadership is to produce more leaders, not more followers." —Ralph Nader

"Leadership is a willingness to take blame." —Joe Montana

"A leader is one who knows the way, goes the way, and shows the way." —John Maxwell

"Why don't I take a step and move forward. When the whole world is silent, even one voice becomes powerful." —Malala Yousafzai

---

While leadership has been defined in many ways (see Box 4.1), it is generally exemplified in five primary areas in palliative care (Dahlin et al., 2019) (see Box 4.2).

BOX 4.2

EXEMPLIFYING LEADERSHIP IN THE PALLIATIVE CARE SETTING

While there are a multitude of ways in which leadership can be enacted in the five dimensions described in the following list, some common scenarios are presented. It is also important to recognize palliative care providers often embody a number of these leadership dimensions simultaneously, and therefore, these dimensions should not be considered as mutually exclusive.

1. **Leadership in Clinical Practice:** In reviewing patient records, a pharmacist may suggest a revised care plan that addresses all of the patient's medical needs, but through fewer or more cost-effective treatment methods.

2. **Leadership in Research:** A palliative care nurse has successfully set up a high-performing interdisciplinary care team. Through case studies, interviews, and observations, she publishes research on best practices for interdisciplinary PCTs to generate evidence-based outcomes for other units and providers.

3. **Leadership in Education and Outreach:** A social worker recognizes a trend among new admits from the same oncology practice. Referrals from this practice are under the impression that they are "building strength" before being referred back to their attending physician. However, in these cases, the social worker has recognized that these patients are no longer responding to curative treatment. As a means to enhance the patient experience and minimize confusion, the social worker schedules meetings with the practice to discuss effective communication strategies for this patient population.

4. **Leadership in Advocacy and Policy:** A chaplain may feel strongly about expanding the reach and patient access to palliative care. He may work with lobbyists or other advocacy groups to consider how to make palliative care a service covered by all insurance providers including Medicare and Medicaid.

5. **Leadership in Administration:** A nurse or physician who has demonstrated success in building or managing a successful practice may be approached to apply those administrative skills (e.g., marketing, scheduling, billing, delivery of care) to the development of a new palliative care unit.

Considering the scope of leadership in palliative care, the importance of effective team leadership is hard to overstate (Omilion-Hodges & Baker, 2017). Those in leadership positions influence other members both directly (through providing instruction and assigning specific responsibilities) and indirectly (by modeling desired team behaviors). Of the four primary threats to palliative care team health identified by Stevens and Reifsnyder (2018), one is specific to leadership and the other three are directly influenced by team leadership.

Threat #1.   Interpersonal communication:

        Lack of trust/collaboration

        Conflict avoidance/poor conflict resolution

Threat #2.   Structural threats:

        Minimal team contact

Threat #3.   Work demands:

     Volume/hours/cases
     Limited support

Threat #4.   Leadership/culture:

     Poorly articulated mission, values, and expectations
     Underestimating process and relationships
     Lack of discipline-specific role clarity
     Lack of recognition of team members' contributions

Given the demand for palliative care and the inherent challenges associated with forming and maintaining healthy teams, awareness of these issues by team leaders is vital. This chapter addresses these challenges in leadership.

Team leaders may encourage and provide members with resources to lead in palliative care through delivering training and engaging in research. As noted in Chapter 3, Formation and Maintenance of High-Performing Palliative Care Teams, team leaders may also reinforce leadership in clinical practice by actively praising members and fostering an environment where members have opportunities to engage in clinical and non–work-related talk. In this sense, team leaders define and reinforce team culture, exemplify the way that members interact with and treat each other, and set standards for patient care. Leaders also impact PCT members' earning potential and promotions via annual reviews and are often tasked with distributing group resources (training dollars, conference funding, etc.) at their discretion.

Another unique element of leadership in palliative care is the assumption that formal leaders (those with the manager, director, or supervisor title) will create an environment of shared leadership. This means that every member, regardless of specialty or seniority level, is expected to exemplify leadership skills in the form of personal accountability and responsibility to their team and in the delivery of patient-centered care. Additionally, as Dahlin et al. (2019) point out, palliative care providers and leaders are accountable for the triple aim initiative of lowering costs, improving the health of populations through better outcomes, and enhancing the patient care experience.

An example of shared leadership through engaged problem-solving is offered in Exhibit 4.1. This PCT is staffed by physicians, APRNs, RN, social workers, chaplains, and a pharmacist, and this conversation came about as a side note during morning table rounds, also known as patient coordination meetings or huddles. This example gets to one of the fundamental issues of the hospital PCT—a team can have highly competent and caring members who work well together, but if they cannot get referrals, they cannot fulfill their goals. This particular team has a large census, but they are also concerned about the unmet palliative care needs they know to exist at their hospital. Since PCTs are dependent on other departments for referrals, the full team engages in a problem-solving process. Throughout this example, both formal leadership and informal leadership are apparent, as a brief interaction description leads the team to talk about a larger problem.

EXHIBIT 4.1

AN EXAMPLE OF LEADING AND PROBLEM-SOLVING DURING A PALLIATIVE CARE TEAM MEETING

APRN1: I can't find this patient. I was like staring at this all last night, so no, she wasn't on the list.

APRN2: Do you think that is the one who said, "No?" Did you call the doctor?

APRN1: That is a nonstarter for me, because there has to be ownership and Dr. Edwards actually said, "It seems like it doesn't make sense for somebody who is not staff on 2 North to be trolling through charts, trying to find people with advanced cancer. Don't the nurses already know that? Why is somebody who doesn't know these patients spending time looking through these things?" So he acknowledged that it's not sustainable and it's dumb. That's basically what he nicely said.

Chaplain: But that's what we are trying to fix!

APRN1: Yeah. The problem is, there is nobody who wants to identify the patients. Nobody wants to follow up. Nobody wants to accept. And then, even if they did, we don't have the staff on PCT for all of them. So what are we doing? There are a lot of barriers to them identifying possible palliative consults, but they weren't quite ready to let go of us completely. In the end, Edwards said, "What if the trigger was just advanced cancer? Stage 4? Surely during huddles that could be identified without PCT being here." And I said, "Hmm, okay." So I gave it up. I'm not going to be tracking anymore.

Physician: But I don't understand how that changes the ultimate problem?

APRN1: It doesn't. If they identify with their own unit staff, then who makes the call to make sure there's a referral? Edwards thinks they should tell the charge nurses to call the doctors.

Social Worker: Mm-hmm, the same charge nurses who are fighting with the nursing supervisor every day to get nurses borrowed from other units, because they don't have enough nurses to staff?

APRN2:	Uh-huh, yeah. That's not going to go well. And then the doctor says, "No, thank you. I don't want to refer." And then, even if they say yes, then we can't actually handle it because of our census and we won't know this is coming.
RN:	The charge nurse is not going to want to take that on. They're down to 13 nurses on day shift staff. They need eight to run the unit on any given day. They're getting called in every time they're on a day off, so those nurses are working eight and nine days in a row.
Physician:	Is there a way to trigger consults on the electronic medical record? I know that would take forever to do, but is that something they could build?
APRN1:	We talked about that with the IT guy there in oncology, and he said we could pilot that, but it can only be cancer patients because that is who he is assigned to. And then I kind of went back to, "Well, that's great, but we don't currently have a staff to handle it anyway." Edwards, I think, has a sort of a visceral reaction against best-practice alerts. It's like ugh—I think they just hate it.
Physician:	What if their negative reaction is about a full consult? Is there way to think about less than a full consult, as a first step? Would that be less intimidating?
Chaplain:	Call it a "Meet and greet" with a "You'll be seeing us again!" Like a social support introduction?
APRN1:	I might come back to that if we find that we're just not keeping up.
Physician:	The other way to think about less threatening ways to help patients is this idea that's emerging with the discharge plan for Javier today.
Social Worker:	That's actually what they want us for—to do this discharge.
Physician:	So, would it make sense to have a social worker not on our team, but a social worker who knows us very well and is more attuned to all of the options for patients and can introduce palliative care in a very cogent, sensitive manner to patients as part of the work of an dedicated discharge planner? Then the ideas are there, but it isn't on our census, and it's not on our social workers' plates—those plates are already full.
Social Worker:	Uh-huh, yeah.
Physician:	Just an idea. We're at a point where we could teach and coach a handful of folks outside of the team who are linked and who are a gateway into a full consult. I mean, it would be hard to imagine the docs routinely turning down dedicated discharge planning for advanced cancer patients. But they'd have to find a way to pay for that person.

Exhibit 4.1 shows an example of useful problem-solving that occurred outside of a stated meeting to solve this particular issue. If team leadership had insisted that the group stay focused only on discussing the patients, this particular systemic problem might not have been noted. This team agrees to allow for short conversations that are on-topic but not specific to the patient for the purpose of identifying issues like these. They manage to stay on schedule by appointing a timekeeper to move the meeting along when necessary.

Exhibit 4.1 is just one example of how formal and informal leadership can function in teams. This section builds on the previous teamwork development section to nuance the role of team leaders. In addition to discussing the structural and relational role expectations of team leaders, suggestions are provided to help new or seasoned team leaders enhance their skills via intentional communication practices.

Importance of Team Leaders

In a perfect world, team leaders would develop and maintain high-quality exchange relationships with each member. These relationships would rest on a foundation of trust, mutual respect, and two-way communication between leader and member. However, because a leader's time and energy are finite and because leaders are people with individual preferences and tendencies, those in formal managerial positions develop relationships of varying quality with each team member. This can stem from gender or personality differences or issues stemming from liking certain team members more than others (Bernerth, Armenakis, Feild, Giles, & Walker, 2007; Varma & Stroh, 2001; Wayne, Shore, & Liden, 1997).

However, it has been suggested (Omilion-Hodges & Baker, 2013, 2017) that if leaders value the collective performance and functioning of their team, they should focus on three priorities:

1. **Managing relationships**

    Relationships are at the heart of leadership. In identifying the 10 most influential priorities for an effective interdisciplinary team, the characteristic at the top of the list was appointing a formal leader who could set a clear vision for the team and orchestrate that vision through adept communication skills: listening, supporting members, providing guidance, and articulating expectations (Nancarrow et al., 2013). This finding shows the dual duty administrative and clinical leaders carry—they are expected to help teams to fulfill organizational goals while also developing individual relationships with each member.

■ **Reflecting on personal tendencies and preferences:** Leaders have to be aware of their own preferences and tendencies because research shows that those in formal leadership positions are not immune to favoritism and may not naturally treat all PCT members equally (Omilion-Hodges & Baker, 2017). Leaders must be aware of the time they spend with each PCT member, how they approach conversations differently with each individual, and how their interactions (positive and negative) with individuals may be interpreted by other team members.

■ **Perception questions about the leader–member relationship:** Attentive leaders work hard to develop team members, and they may wonder how individual leader–member relationships are perceived by others. Asking a close friend or romantic partner for their perceptions of these relationships is a good way to find out. It is likely that either over dinner or while venting about work, team leaders provide clues about which of their work relationships are easier or more challenging to manage. If others are able to pick up on these clues, it can be assumed that team members are also well aware of them.

■ **Consider the channel of communication used to communicate dissent:** Turnage and Goodboy (2016) discovered the willingness to use email to communicate dissent was a reliable indicator of leader–member status. Team members are willing to articulate dissent in face-to-face communication if they perceive a good relationship with the supervisor. They are also more likely to do so if they find that as a team member, their solutions are considered competent so they are willing to subject the ideas to constructive criticism. If the team member feels a high degree of trust with the team, email will also be utilized because the members do not worry about creating a written record that may be held against them. However, outgroup members are more likely to email people in leadership positions as the computer "acts as a shield" (p. 279).

2. **Managing resources**

Leaders are often charged with managing and being a good steward of the team's resources. These resources are most often considered monetary, yet resource types surpass managing merit raises and equipment budgets. Leaders have a variety of positive and negative resources at their disposal, and the way that these resources are often exchanged from leader to member is in the form of verbal and nonverbal communication. There are a number of ways in which a leader can interact with members to provide instruction, maintain relationships, and collaborate for patient care. Some of these communicative changes can be inherently positive, whereas others may be perceived as negative.

■ Positive resources are typically desired and enjoyed by members with whom the leader has a high-quality relationship (see Box 4.3 for tips on leader–member relationship development).

BOX 4.3

HOW DO LEADER–MEMBER RELATIONSHIP DEVELOP?

Phase 1—Role Taking: When you join a new team, your leader is assessing how well you are completing your tasks and how well you are fitting into the workgroup. You are also getting to know your leader, and he or she is getting to know you—so you may find you are observing each other and trying to figure out how each other prefer to communicate.

Angela, RN (upon hire): When I first started, my lead was really clear that the first thing I needed to do was learn my core responsibilities. I worked off checklists, and she looked in on my progress about once a week to make sure I was getting the hang of things. Once in a while, we would talk about other ways to expand my role on the team—we called it the "Angela Expansion List"—but we agreed it was important to nail down the basics of triage and documentation first.

Phase 2—Role Making: If you demonstrate a satisfactory or better grasp of role-related tasks, your leader will typically allow you some flexibility to mold the position into one that highlights your strengths. This phase is characterized by trust building and a lot of communicative exchange in the form of negotiation and give and take between you and your leader.

Angela, RN (after 3 months): Once I was able to effectively coordinate the team, we went back to our list of ideas to improve care. I had some background in the ICU so we decided it would be a great idea for me to start attending their rounds a couple of days a week. It's been great because I've been able to improve communication between our teams and identify patients who should be referred earlier. So now, I'm adding value to the team that wasn't there before.

Phase 3—Role Routinization: Routinization details an established leader–member relationship. This relationship can be an effective, high-quality relationship or one that lacks trust and is transactional in nature. It is always more advantageous for PCT members to develop high-quality relationships because they often come with greater access to positive resources and opportunities.

Angela, RN (after 1 year): I know my job well now, and I look for ways on my own to make this team function better. I've brought a fresh perspective to the role and my lead trusts me to find new ways to improve patient care. She has been able to let go of some the tasks she used to have to manage because she knows that I've got it taken care of.

2. **Managing resources** (continued)

Recent communication scholarship (Omilion-Hodges & Baker, 2017) verified six dimensions of positive leader communication exchange including:

1. Behaviors that indicate the PCT member has the leader's *professional trust* (see Box 4.4)

2. Leader actions, such as personal mentoring, that demonstrate the leader is invested in the PCT member's *professional development*

3. *Affective* managerial behavior that demonstrates care or concern

4. Positive *verbal exchanges*, such as the team leader praising the PCT member

5. *Nonverbal affirmation* from the team leader such as open body language and eye contact

6. The leader makes himself or herself *accessible* to PCT members

Negative resources describe leader–member interactions that are not necessarily desirable, but may leave the PCT member feeling left out or as if their leader does not trust them or their professional abilities.

BOX 4.4

CHECKING EGOS AHEAD OF TIME

We really try to check our egos ahead of time. So that really helps us avoid negative conflict. Decision-making is approached with "I'm the point person on this team, but what are we going to do now? Am I still the right person?" I may get assigned a case, and when I look into it, I might say "You know what? Maybe this is better handled by the chaplain." We might say "Let's bring this back. Maybe we are having trouble on this case because it's the wrong person taking the lead."—Roger, PCT physician

The same research that statistically validated dimensions of positive resources also uncovered negative dimensions:

1. In place of opportunities to learn more, a leader may restrict or block an associate's *professional development*.

2. Leaders may also exclude certain PCT members from informal gatherings, such as lunch invitations, or from *social* conversations.

3. *Betrayal* of a PCT member's confidence or reporting an associate to upper management without first addressing the concern with the PCT member.

4. Leaders may unknowingly belittle PCT members' ideas or critique their work in public or through an unnecessarily harsh lens indicating little to no *professional trust*.

5. Team leaders may not indicate respect to PCT members through their *verbal communication* such as in the form of interrupting them or reacting before considering the consequences.

6. Those in formal leadership positions may demonstrate negative *nonverbal communication* actions by not listening to PCT members or giving what are perceived as "dirty looks."

Since it is hard to develop trust if team members do not perceive that the leader is fully present when they are in conversation together, it is time to put the phone down. In the fast-paced day of hospital care, cell phones and other devices for communicating and interacting with electronic medical records are simply a part of the workplace. However, if team leaders use such devices during interpersonal interactions (e.g., answering a text while simultaneously having a conversation with a colleague about how to work with a patient), the use of the device may negatively impact their perceived immediacy. While people often think of themselves as competent multitaskers and devices influence that perception of ability, it is difficult to be perceived as fully present when a device is

BOX 4.5

PROJECTING PRESENCE THROUGH IMMEDIACY BEHAVIORS
Convincing Colleagues That You Are Present in the Conversation

Alfred Mehrabian (1981) studied nonverbal behaviors in majority Western cultures and their influence on perception. *Immediacy behaviors* are those that are perceived as communicative openness by conversational partners. These behaviors signify investment and attentiveness to the interaction. In mainstream Western cultures, nonverbal immediacy behaviors include:

- Attentive body orientation (e.g., turning to face the other person)
- Closer distance
- Slight forward lean of upper body
- Eye contact
- Open and relaxed postures

SOURCE: Mehrabian, A. (1981). *Silent messages: Implicit communication of emotions and attitudes.* Belmont, CA: Wadsworth Publishing Company

in the mix. What seems like a timesaver may be negatively impacting collegial relationships and may cost team leaders' credibility and increase team turnover (Kelly & Westerman, 2014; Lybarger, Rancer, & Lin, 2017).

Immediacy behaviors are those that communicate that a person is there in the moment with a conversational partner. Immediacy behaviors in Western mainstream cultures include actions such as those in Box 4.5 (Mehrabian, 1981). These behaviors are usually received as signals of approachability, liking, and involvement. A study by Kelly and Westerman (2014) found that when supervisor immediacy behaviors were perceived by subordinates as an interaction in which the supervisor was fully present and invested, the subordinates scored lower on burnout measures. They also found positive relationships between supervisor immediacy behaviors and employee motivation, empowerment, and job satisfaction.

Lybarger et al. (2017) experimented to see if nonverbal immediacy could moderate verbal aggression in communication from superiors to subordinates. While they found that those performing immediacy behaviors without verbally aggressive messages were "perceived as being significantly more competent, significantly higher in character, and significantly more caring" (p. 131), they also found that superiors performing immediacy behavior paired with verbal aggression scored lowest on competency. Applied to PCTs, team leaders would be wise to remember that many of their colleagues are highly attuned to their nonverbal behaviors. If a team lead is performing "I'm present in this conversation" behaviors such as a slight forward lean and appropriate eye contact but is also verbally berating a team member, the leader will be seen as less competent. If the lead needs to give corrective feedback to a colleague, the colleague is mostly likely to be able to hear and process that correction if the team lead performs immediacy nonverbal behaviors paired with a message that is assertive in content and lacks any personal attacks.

Finally, attempting to communicate immediacy will fail if it is paired with simultaneous work on a phone or another electronic device. If it is necessary to respond to a text or answer a phone call while in conversation with a team member, excuse yourself from the conversation and answer. This is the ultimate timesaver—while it may seem that answering the message while in conversation with others is efficient, doing so can decrease efficiency as you will need to ask for repeated information and you may miss the emotional content of the message from the first time it was communicated. Decreasing your ability to communicate immediacy to your team also decreases your interpersonal effectiveness and will cost you time in the long run as you attempt to strengthen or rebuild connection with your team.

When professional trust exists, team leaders can address leadership decisions and team decisions with a constructive critical eye. If the team does not trust one another, such criticism is met with defensiveness, and opportunities for course corrections are lost. When teams develop professional trust and become comfortable in the interdisciplinary model, conversations such as those in Box 4.6 are possible.

BOX 4.6

MODELING INTENTIONAL COMMUNICATION: LEARNING TO HANDLE THE OVERLAP

Cara, a nurse, and Sarie, a social worker, experienced some transdisciplinary tension early in their tenure of working together. Cara is often seen as a communication leader on this team. Sarie reflects on their interaction:

It was a compliment, really. I mean, we spend so much time together that Cara learned a lot of the things I do. And then when we met with the family, she told them the things the nurse usually covers but when they asked a hospice placement question, she went ahead and answered it. She gave them the right information, but it meant that I was like "Oh, so you are going to do that. So what do I do now?" When we left the family I said to her "It's okay if you want to share that information, but that means you really don't need me in there. If that's what you want, fine, but don't take me along to the meeting if I'm not going to have anything to do." Then she said "Oh! Sorry, I'm a talker, and I just kept talking. I'll watch that" and I thought "Okay, I think we are going to work together well."

Sarie's response belied the truth that she was more upset than she wanted people to know. Cara's response took responsibility for her actions and calmed Sarie's concerns of inadequacy and invisibility in the group. Sarie says that in a different group, she would be concerned that people thought she was not necessary at her job, and she might not have believed a response like Cara gave. However, her high degree of trust in her team members and her belief that every person on the team works here because they are kind and caring people allowed her to receive Cara's apology as sincere.

3. Managing perceptions of relationships and resources

Considering the interdependence among members in a true interdisciplinary care team coupled with the fact that there has been a 50% increase in the amount of time leaders and members spend in collaboration over the past two decades (Cross, Rebele, & Grant, 2016), many PCT members are in a position to evaluate and compare their leader–member relationship with that of their peers (Box 4.7).

BOX 4.7

WAIT! THE RELATIONSHIP I HAVE WITH MY LEADER IMPACTS MY PEER RELATIONSHIPS?

Do you really dislike your team leader or maybe you have never connected?

While this may be the case, it is in your best interest (in most cases) to be flexible and consider how to strengthen the relationship you share with your leader.

Why? Research (Baker & Omilion-Hodges, 2014; Omilion-Hodges & Baker, 2017; Sherony & Green, 2002) continues to show a link between leader–member relationships and the development of peer relationships.

Members who share high-quality relationships with the leader are more likely to befriend and exchange with one another. This means that those who have access to more positive resources such as professional development opportunities are also more likely to share trusting relationships with peers who also have high-quality relationships with the leader. This substantially increases these PCT members' access to information, mentoring, and social support at work.

Members who have a lower quality or strained relationship with the team leader tend to not only have a compromised relationship with their leader, but also with their team members who have strong leader-member relationships. This means that they are not only likely to be the recipients of a leader's negative resources, but they will also likely develop their strongest working relationships with other members in similar relationship to the leader (who also have restricted access to positive resources).

SOURCE: Baker, C. R., & Omilion-Hodges, L. M. (2014). The effect of leader-member exchange differentiation within work units on coworker exchange and organizational citizenship behaviors. *Communication Research Reports, 30*, 313–322. doi:10.1080/08824096.2013.837387; Omilion-Hodges, L. M., & Baker, C. R. (2017). Communicating leader-member relationship quality: The development of leader communication exchange scales to measure relationship building and maintenance through the exchange of communication-based goods. *International Journal of Business Communication, 54*(2), 115–145. doi:10.1177/2329488416687052; Sherony, K. M., & Green, S. G. (2002). Coworker exchange: Relationships between coworkers, leader-member exchange, and work attitudes. *Journal of Applied Psychology, 87*, 542–548. doi:10.1037/0021-9010.87.3.542

An important leadership role on PCTs is serving as a liaison to the larger hospital in which the PCT is embedded. The hospital ultimately controls the resources and processes of the PCT, and it remains true that not all hospital administrators will understand the PCT's function for patients and families or how the PCT can save the hospital money.

One of the language cues that there are concerns or challenges with perceptions of the larger organization within which the PCT is housed is a referral to organizational "politics." When members are planning to make a move to a new organization, they are often heard to exclaim "I can't wait to get out of here and away from all the politics!" A reasonable answer to this statement is "Oh, so you plan to be self-employed?" because organizational politics is a fact of organizations. When people express the desire to get away from workplace politics, they hope to escape the seemingly endless jockeying for position that occurs as a part of most places of work. That jockeying occurs at the interpersonal level with power hierarchies, personality differences, and different ideas about how individual positions contribute to the team. These politics also occur between the team and its larger organization. The politics a team member may plan to flee are the politics of this particular organization. The next organization the team member joins will surely have its own set of politics that will become clear over time.

These politics bear investigating because they are indicators of how organizations and teams think about team identity, and part of the job of PCT leadership is to facilitate that identity within the team and between the team and the organization. Payne (2006) defines identity politics in interaction with teams with multiple disciplines as "a joint negotiation of meaning about the contributions that different professionals make to a specialized community of practice" (p. 138). While many think of identity as what teams decide to be, identity is formed, in part, through this joint meaning-making process.

Power is always an issue in politics, and when it comes to identity politics, personal and group identity is certainly affected by power. Due to the complex nature of organizations, a person at a high level of administration who is relatively unconnected with a group or specialty may be defining that group in a way that is not consistent with how the PCT practices (Payne, 2006). It can be a difficult organizational shift from "hospitals as places of curing" to "hospitals as places of caring" in which curing is a very important factor but not the only factor considered for caring. When those with powerful voices in hospitals are against this shift, they may talk about, and therefore construct, the identity of PCTs as the people you see when "you give up" or when medicine "fails." This construction of the PCT allows for the dominant voices to diminish the importance and the professionalism of palliative care providers.

Identity politics is also at play between the hospital in which the PCT operates and accrediting organizations. For example, as established in Chapter 3, Formation and Maintenance of High-Performing Palliative Care Teams, high-performing teams require extensive coordination, trust, and power sharing. Yet, the effectiveness of the team is never the only criterion for success as the professional disciplines, to which each team member belongs, all have their own set of rules and structures. The ability to follow those rules and structures is also a part of how a team is assessed; those external structures play a defining role in the identity of the team even if they move the team away from what the team finds to be most effective. Finding the balance between team identity based on its experiential knowledge and outside agency requirements for that team can be a true leadership challenge. For example, to achieve Magnet® status, an accreditation awarded by the American Nurses Credentialing Center (ANCC), hospitals must have an organizational structure where nurses report to nurses with the same or a higher level of education as they have. A team may consider its interdisciplinary or even trans-disciplinary identity as one that has moved beyond traditional power structures to be highly effective for patient and family care. Yet, to align with the hospital's strategic plan (such as achieving Magnet® status), the team's reporting structure may also need to conform with existing organizational hierarchies (Figure 4.1A).

Additionally, the health system of billing and revenue generation places an artificial structure on PCTs where billing and nonbilling healthcare professionals reside in separate organizational entities (Figure 4.1B). Navigating this organizational structure is required for teams to gain the resources they need to do their work, but it also imposes an extra level of difficulty for leadership. One PCT lead said "I tried to put our organizational chart down on paper and I failed. I couldn't do it. I may be the team lead but I'm not the medical director. And while I'm the team lead, the various members of our team also have their own discipline-specific reporting structure." Even for cohesive teams that believe all team members are equally important, conflict can arise based on the actual hierarchies of reporting structures and the implied hierarchies based on who provides services for which the hospital codes and bills and who does not.

Payne (2006) also reminds us that identities are constructed through differentiating themselves from others. In palliative care, this part of identity politics may seem more apparent, as PCTs position themselves as a subspecialty (caring without necessarily curing) and by their team type (interdisciplinary and so not constrained by silos). Even as a team solidifies good practices for themselves, it may take some time for other hospital departments to buy in, so the kneejerk reaction may be to resist or decline help from a PCT. This is more likely if accepting the PCT's help means that the department has to let go of something they have been doing themselves, regardless of how well they were doing it. Even though having

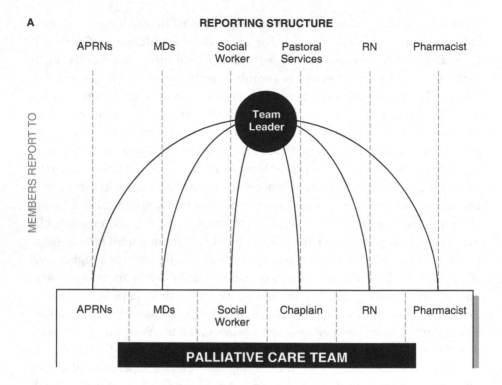

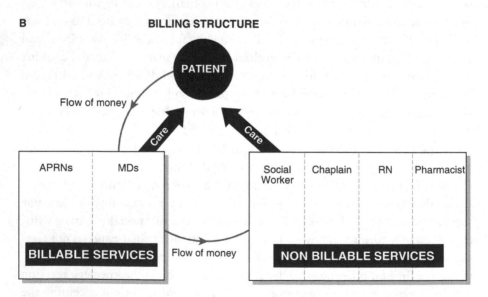

FIGURE 4.1 (A) Hospital reporting structures. (B) Hospital billing structures.

the PCT involved may help that department's workload and positively impact the care of patients and families, the identity politics make it seem that accepting help means losing something. Overcoming these reactions will take time. If possible, leaders should approach members of other departments who seem willing to talk and try to drill down to the ultimate source of the resistance. Asking "Why?" can help uncover those reasons. The first two or three answers to "Why?" may still be on the surface of the problem, but repeated questioning can unearth the identity politics such as the following:

- I'm worried our department will lose money or positions to your team.
- I'm anxious that allowing your department to help will make me or my department seem less competent.
- I'm concerned that your help might make my job irrelevant.

It takes a skillful communicator and a high degree of trust to uncover these types of self-disclosures, and it may take multiple interactions to reach this depth.

A Mark of a Successful Team Leader

Concerned about how to manage the role responsibilities that come with being a team lead coupled with the challenges that come from relationships and resources? A leader's true success may emerge from intentional and reflective communication practices. That is, a successful team leader may best lead the team by regularly reflecting on how the leader relates to each member, how this is demonstrated in the workplace, and how members may interpret and react to the varied distribution of a leader's resources. The following section provides some practical tips and suggestions for current team leaders and for those who aspire to formal leadership in the future.

Modeling Intentional, Relational Communication Within the Team

Leadership is in the eye of the beholder. This is helpful for team leaders, as they are able to communicate differently based on each member's needs and preferences. For example, a new team member may need more attention and mentoring from the team leader, whereas the leader can convey his or her trust in seasoned members by giving them latitude to fulfill their responsibilities as they see fit. This is what is meant by communicating like a leader—taking the time to reflect on each member's needs and then communicating in ways that validate and fulfill those needs. Leadership is not a one-size-fits-all endeavor, but intentional, relationship-based communication helps those in formal leadership positions to develop high-quality relationships with each member. For teams that desire to move beyond interdisciplinary to transdisciplinary teams, building and maintaining trust is essential. Maintenance of good communication practices is necessary in all relationships, and that is particularly true for those who want to transition to the transdisciplinary team model. These teams require a high frequency and high volume of communication. One way that PCTs can facilitate frequent and successful communication is through structured team meetings. Chapter 5, Interdisciplinary Palliative Care Team Meetings, focuses on this aspect of task-related communication via team meetings. Task-related communication is the most likely content of this communication, but for transdisciplinary teams to work, regular relationship communication is essential. Even a team with high trust will need to continually discuss what it means to be on this team.

Communicating Like a Leader

Just as developing competency and comfort in communicating effectively with seriously ill patients takes practice, reflection, and some instruction, communicating as a leader requires the same level of intentionality. This is a learnable skill. Here are three guiding principles to help new leaders and to remind experienced leaders of best practices.

1. **Relationships Come First:** Without the buy-in and trust of members, an individual's tenure in a leadership role is limited. Leadership is challenging in any context but may be especially so in the case of interdisciplinary teams. In PCTs, leaders must be mindful to validate the training and expertise of individual members, while also promoting an environment of interdependence, flexibility, and collaborative leadership (Gray, 2008). This means discarding antiquated authoritative ways to embrace the notion that all members are responsible for demonstrating leadership. This may be in the form of speaking up and offering a novel solution or in voicing a potential consequence that has not yet been considered. This may also present by members taking a step back and giving other team members the space to offer suggestions or devise care plans.

   As Table 4.1 shows, focusing on relationships often feels like a luxury— something you only do when everything is going well. While Table 4.1 does illustrate when it is easiest to focus on relationships, that focus is important at all times lest the team fail to function as a collective and revert to a loosely connected group of individual professionals. While interdisciplinary teams are the current gold standard of palliative care, they are not easy to establish. The move to create transdisciplinary teams will create even more challenges as, in that model, role blurring is normative and helpful rather than confusing and threatening. However, given the potential gains for patient and

TABLE 4.1 **Focusing on Relationships in Teams**

FOCUSING ON RELATIONSHIPS FIRST IS EASY WHEN ...	FOCUSING ON RELATIONSHIPS FIRST IS CHALLENGING WHEN ...
The team has a clear goal, purpose, and member buy-in.	Lacking a clear and shared purpose, members revert to providing care as individual practitioners instead of as a holistic care team.
Team members have clearly defined individual roles and understand how their roles interact and overlap with other members. This gives the team added bench strength as members know who else, if necessary, can fulfill similar duties if necessary.	Members do not support the shared team purpose. In some cases, members are assigned into palliative care teams by administration, or members take a position until they feel that something more suitable opens up.
Team members value the contributions of each other.	Members are overworked or understaffed. Palliative care is challenging in and of itself, but the emotional labor increases if patient census is too high or if the PCT is understaffed for long periods of time. This can also lead to compassion fatigue and/ or provider burnout (Back, Steinhauser, Kamal, & Johnson, 2016).
Team members have identified parameters or best practices for handling conflict.	The team leader does not personally like or get along with a member.
Team members know each other as people. Sharing lunch, a coffee break, or an occasional drink outside of work may help members to work together more cohesively in their delivery of patient-centered care.	
The team has a consistent, yet manageable, patient census and access to all of the resources, including enough providers, to meet patient needs.	
The team feels that members are supported by administration.	

SOURCE: From Back, A. L., Steinhauser, K. E., Kamal, A. H., & Jackson, V. A. (2016). Building resilience for palliative care clinicians: An approach to burnout prevention based on individual skills and workplace factors. *Journal of Pain and Symptom Management, 52*(2), 284–291. doi:10.1016/j.jpainsymman.2016 .02.002; Dahlin, C., Coyne, P., Goldberg, J., & Vaughan, L. (2019). Palliative care leadership. *Journal of Palliative Care, 34*, 21–28. doi:10.1177/0825859718791427; Nancarrow, S. A., Booth, A., Ariss, S., Smith, T., Enderby, P., & Roots, A. (2013). Ten principles of good interdisciplinary team work. *Human Resources for Health, 11*, 11–19. doi:10.1186/1478-4491-11-19; Omilion-Hodges, L. M., & Baker, C. R. (2017). Communicating leader-member relationship quality: The development of leader communication exchange scales to measure relationship building and maintenance through the exchange of communication-based goods. *International Journal of Business Communication, 54*(2), 115–145. doi:10.1177/2329488416687052

family care and team health, striving to create these types of teams is a worthy endeavor for PCTs.

Many of the challenges for focusing on relationships in teams are related to the difficulties of managing a complex team as a part of a complex organization. Issues of adequate resources for staffing, making time to get to know one another as individuals, and working through the constraints imposed by the larger organization can be time-consuming for problem-solving and frustrating for day-to-day team functioning. The team leader faces a specific facilitation challenge if a member or members reject team norms such as the way they adhere to handling conflict and approaches to patient care, or neglect to treat members with respect.

While the complexity of PCTs in the context of the complexity of the hospital lends itself to a number of leadership challenges, one of the harder challenges for leaders to navigate is not an organizational challenge at all. Team leaders are people like everyone else. This means that they may foster their own preferences and tendencies and may find themselves in a position where it is challenging to work with a certain individual for a variety of reasons. As noted in the managing relationships section, team leaders should reflect on their individual leader–member relationships and consider why some are stronger than others. As an additional note, it is particularly important that team leaders (and all organizational members for that matter) are aware of any certain prejudices they may foster and ensure that they are not discriminating against a member unlawfully.

2. **Transparency Is Key:** Committing to transparent communication seems easy, yet it often goes against instinctual decision-making because the information provided may upset some members. Remember, the purpose of organizational transparency is not to make people happy; the purpose is to provide information so members can make informed decisions. Omilion-Hodges and Baker (2014) found that even distressing news, such as budget cuts, can be palatable when it is communicated clearly and early. While not every member will likely earn the same performance bonus or merit raise and some members will earn praise and promotion more quickly than others, it is the leader's responsibility to articulate expectations and to tie high-quality work to rewards. Team leaders begin to set a precedent in acknowledging members who provide exemplary care or commitment to the team. In these cases, team leaders should do more than just to say "good work" but rather use the opportunity to highlight the specifics of the job well done. By doing so, the nuances of exemplary work are clear to all members. Relatedly, when an individual is promoted, rewarded with a bonus,

or granted funding to attend a conference, it does not feel like a mystery or decision that took place in a black box. Committing to clearly articulating why decisions are made and how resources are disseminated promotes a culture of equity, which in turn leads to stronger team and peer relationships (Omilion-Hodges & Baker, 2013).

Part of creating transparency is helping people to understand the "why" of a decision. To cultivate a culture of transparency, be very careful with using the phrase *I can't* as an explanation. *I can't* is useful for showing a lack of capacity (e.g., "*I can't* draw a blood sample because I do not have the training to do so.") or an organizational or policy constraint (e.g., "*I can't* get your sister a bed at that hospice because she does not meet the criteria for that facility."). If leaders hide behind "*I can't*" when what they really mean is "*We decided not to…*" or "*I don't want to…*," team members are prevented from joining the meaning-making process in a useful way.

Psychologist Heidi Grant Halvorson thinks about these phrases in terms of motivating personal decisions saying, "*I don't* is experienced as a choice, so it feels empowering. *I can't* isn't a choice—it's a restriction, it's being imposed upon you … *I can't* undermines your sense of power and personal agency" (2013). While these phrases impact personal thinking about the willingness and ability to act, they also impact team members who hear them as explanations for decision-making. The desire to blame institutional rules or policies with *I can't* may be strong because then team members can be annoyed or angry with the organization and the leader might avoid an unpleasant interpersonal interaction. However, the conclusion of one interaction is always the starting point for the next interaction. If members do not know the true reason for the denial, they will be unable to participate in solving any patterned problems around this issue. If and when it comes out that the real answer was *I won't* rather than *I can't*, trust in leadership is inevitably damaged. Intentional use of *I don't* or *I won't* with appropriate explanations will also help differentiate dissent from obstruction. Dissent is useful to group decision-making; obstruction is not. Purposeful use of *I can't* and *I won't* can help teams determine whether conflicts are built on dissent or obstruction, allowing leaders and team members to choose wisely in their approach to move on to a solution (Table 4.2).

3. **Role Model Desired Behaviors and Communication Practices:** A true leader should never find himself or herself in a position where he or she has to tell members to "do as I say, not as I do." This would mean that the leader is engaging in behaviors that are contrary to those that are desired or expected. The *I can't* versus *I won't/don't* issue is a specific example of role modeling desired communication practices. It can be frustrating to hear a team member voice "I can't" when the team knows the issue is that the

TABLE 4.2 **Substituting for** *I Can't*

INSTEAD OF:	TRY:	WHY?
We can't hire another dedicated pharmacist because we can't afford it.	*We decided not to hire* another pharmacist at this time. We did consider your argument, and we decided to assign the new personnel line to oncology because of the growth of their patient census and the announcement of an impending retirement.	Issues of personnel resource use is often contentious. When leaders say "I can't hire...," but member see equivalent amounts of money spent elsewhere, the logic doesn't hold up. The requesting department may not be happy to hear another department's needs were of higher priority, but for future requests, they will understand the parameters in which the decisions were made.
I can't switch your schedule.	I appreciate your need for flexibility right now, but *I don't have anyone* to fill in for you. *I don't want to fill in myself* due to my own schedule restraints.	Day-to-day logistics may be flexible until they are not. If leaders have made such arrangements in the past, the person requesting flexibility will be confused by the new seeming inability to do so (I can't.). While it is hard to say to our colleagues, if a leader does not want to do something, it is better to say that than to lean on an imaginary organizational constraint.

member just does not want to. Modeling the communication behaviors as a leader can influence team members to do the same both on this team and in other groups in which they participate.

This is just one aspect of being a leader that is hard. Team leaders are charged with overseeing the collective functioning of the group, developing and maintaining leader–member relationships, and managing team resources, all while delivering exemplary clinical care or administration. Yet, if the team leader is not patient and attentive to members, how can he or she expect members to treat each other with respect? It is recommended that team leaders try to consider how observers would describe their behavior. Are they generous with their time and expertise or do they appear rushed and hurried in their interactions with team members and patients? Do team leaders give members the benefit of the doubt and frame errors or oversights as learning moments instead of mistakes? The more mindful team leaders are of their own communication and relational tendencies, the more they may be able to understand the overall culture and climate of their team (Nancarrow et al., 2013).

Team Growth: Selecting and Orienting New Team Members

When the patient census for the PCT grows and the team can show the hospital how their work increases the quality of patient care while saving the hospital money, the team may receive approval to grow their numbers and hire new team members. The selection of and orientation of these team members is an important step. Regardless of the type of team, orientation is always important. In Box 4.8, one social worker shares what it was like to come to a hospital after years of working in nonprofits outside of a hospital setting.

BOX 4.8

A SOCIAL WORKER REFLECTS ON HOSPITAL ACRONYM SHOCK

When you look at our notes, I think probably the first impression is particularly confusing—"What the hell does this all mean?" in terms of all of these abbreviations. At first, I couldn't even figure out what things meant. This was a whole new language. I don't even think I was looking at the team interpersonally yet; I think I was looking at, "I don't even know what these people are saying." You know, I had some medical social work experience, working *in* mental health and working with Alzheimer's disease, but certainly not to this degree, and then there's so many specialties that we cover. So, it was hospital acronym shock.

The social worker's challenge of orienting to the language and customs of a hospital environment include some of the easier orientation points for team leads to remember. However, health practitioners, such as nurses, may also need orientation to the team. PCTs may forget what it is like to work on more teams that are not interdisciplinary and therefore may inadvertently expect new team members to orient faster than is reasonable given the change that they are experiencing in both team and organizational culture. In the example in Box 4.9, a nurse new to an established PCT reflects on how her challenges in her new position were primarily about organizational and team culture and communication practices. Even though she was a good fit for the position, it took time to reframe her thinking about how to do her job in this new environment.

BOX 4.9

A NURSE REFLECTS: THIS IS HARDER THAN I THOUGHT IT WOULD BE
I do have a fair amount of experience, but the transition from hospice to inpatient palliative care has been hard. I'd been the hospice liaison for this hospital for three to four years, and working with this team was a great opportunity. But it has been hard to get used to. Initially, I felt overwhelmed at least once a week—it was just so new. You don't know any of the doctors; they don't know you. This hospital is so big to just figure out. The culture in general took a very long time for me. So, there was that learning curve.

And then there was how to approach things. It was a struggle for me initially, coming from a hospice admissions background where my job was to get a plan, activate the plan, tie the plan all up in a bow, and pass it on to somebody else seamlessly. So, I was wanting to tie it all up. I mean, I would say probably my biggest takeaway from this job is that sometimes there isn't a tidy solution. You have to really keep a big picture focus. That patient will probably come in again for the same problem, but they might have a different understanding of their disease and maybe have different goals. So, an ongoing battle for me is to think about palliative care as caring for patients over time, I guess.

Leading Through Team Changes

The stage model in Chapter 3, Formation and Maintenance of High-Performing Palliative Care Teams (Figure 3.2), has arrows connecting all of the stages because teams do not proceed in a linear fashion from beginning to performing and/or ending. A team may observe they have reached the performing stage with a sigh of relief, but even this stage is not stagnant. Team performance levels will ebb and flow even if the team's process does not return to a previous stage. Changes in team membership are likely to signal a change in team development stage, as there will be new people to orient and with whom to work. This is a vital time for leadership to be responsive in their work with the team and intentional in their communication and organizational planning.

Attentiveness in selecting new team members is very important. However, too often, team leadership fails to follow up the investment of time and effort in selection of team members with the same investment to orienting new members. Participation in orienting new members is important for all team members, but, ultimately, it is the responsibility of team leadership to make sure that it happens and that it is effective. Box 4.10 shows how orientation often happens. It is clear that the physician is well intentioned and believes that the clinical fellows will be

BOX 4.10

ORIENTING NEW MEMBERS: CLINICAL FELLOWS

The team embraces each new fellow as another full member of the team. They [the fellows] will spend some time with the social workers to learn that part and with the chaplains to learn that part and with the nurse practitioners to learn their role. But when we divide patients up, the fellows want them and we give them patients for them to take ownership of. And if they get in over their heads, obviously there's other people on the team, so it's easy to help them out. So far, I think that's worked. We haven't had any one just fold. They [fellows] want responsibility and really look forward to the challenges. I think they learn a lot from doing it on their own and getting it right or getting it wrong.—Samar, PCT physician

helped if needed; however, that relies on the fellows to (a) know they need help and (b) ask for help in a timely manner before the situation gets worse. This process can be better when orientation is more than giving a tour of the hospital, meeting with HR, and making sure all team members make the new person feel welcome.

Weick (1995) reminds us that organizations are always creating themselves; they are constantly organizing. This is true for the PCTs as well. Team leaders who are attentive to both the selection of and orienting of team members are more likely to discover unintentionally harmful messages and structures that persist in teams and organizations. The metaphor of a long-used recipe is apt here. A cook makes a dish so frequently that the recipe itself is no longer used because the cook already knows the ingredients and steps. If the cook returns to the original recipe and compares it to how the dish is made now, it is likely that many subtle shifts in ingredient use or amount, baking times, and so on have occurred over time. Likewise, if organizations continue to give the same generic orientation over and over, it is unlikely to match how team members really function from day to day. Yet that generic orientation fixes a structure in the mind of the new member and it will take time to overcome that mindset. Attentiveness to orienting the new member to how the team does work rather than how the team used to work is important. Weick (2005) finds heedful management of orienting is most useful in helping new members to work well with the team and the team to work well with new members. This type of leadership also prepares teams and individuals to handle the unexpected. The ability to handle the unexpected is a hallmark of good teams and is particularly important in working with seriously ill patients and their families.

Teams may think that refilling a position vacated by a member changes the team less than selecting new team members due to team growth. Whatever the reason, selecting and orienting new team members will bring team changes. It falls to the leader to facilitate discussion about the changes and to model desired behaviors (e.g., welcoming a new member, addressing conflict or confusion directly) as well as ensuring that new team member orientation is effective. Some changes, such as having a new personality on the team to get used to, are expected. Other changes are surprising. For example, long-standing team members may find that old inse-curities arise again with a change in team membership. One APRN laughed as she commented that when someone new starts on the team, it is

> *"Everyone's Insecure Month! We laugh about it later. Lots of us have imposter syndrome, you know, feeling like a fraud even though you know you are qualified to do your job? And we think someone is going to find out—particularly when new people join the team."*

She explains that once she was comfortable with the team, her imposter syn-drome feelings lessened, but they return every time a new person joins the team. As part of her orienting role, to encourage the new hire and assure them they are doing well, she finds it particularly funny, in retrospect, that her own insecurities reappear at that time. In situations like this, the leader may decide to start the team meeting with a lighthearted "Welcome to everyone's Insecure Month again." This could be a way to integrate humor while also addressing the recurrent theme the team faces when onboarding a new member. Addressing the situation head on gives members the opportunity to relax and to engage in formal (in team meetings) and informal (over lunch) conversations about how they are making sense of their role in light of their new colleague.

What to Do When a Team Member Is Not a Good Fit

Unfortunately, even a thorough and attentive orientation cannot solve the prob-lem of a team member who is not a good fit. No team is immune from the trou-bles of selecting a new team member who ultimately does not fit with the team. This experience can cause cognitive dissonance for leaders and team members, particularly those who feel that their opinions were taken seriously by a higher-

BOX 4.11

A PCT LEADER REFLECTS: FINDING THE RIGHT PERSON
FOR THE ROLE
We really struggled with our RN coordinator role. As our PCT grew, it was becoming harder and harder to hold everything together without someone coordinating our efforts throughout the day. We were passing the main phone around like a hot potato and

missing urgent calls and new consults. When we first conceived of the idea of hiring a dedicated RN to do things like handling triage, managing data, and mentoring staff, the hospital didn't really have an existing job code for the role. We got it funded but we had to shoehorn the role into a job description and title that didn't actually fit our needs. The applicant pool was drawn to the idea of doing a lot of direct palliative care work rather than the day to day coordination that we needed. Even though we tried to be clear about the role during interviews, the RN we hired never really took to it. We did a lot of coaching and tried all sorts of things to make it work, including actually reorganizing how the team functioned in order to find ways to give the new hire more of the direct patient care she craved. It was frustrating because, even though technically we had a person to handle the core responsibilities we'd envisioned, the reality was that she was so involved with patient care that she didn't have time to coordinate our team. Ultimately, it just became clear it wasn't going to work and she left the position. It was painful for everyone—it felt like we failed. Afterward, we went back to the drawing board and reimagined the role. Our leadership was able to get approval for a job title and description that matched our needs, and we tailored our interview questions to find an RN who was a good fit.

level administrative leader and that those opinions were carefully discerned based on the person's abilities and potential fit for the group. When someone is not a good fit, it feels like a failure for the team (Box 4.11). Feelings of failure can cause teams to retain a problematic team member long after coaching attempts fail.

Managing Team Outcomes

In addition to the management of interpersonal relationships in the team and team resources, the importance of outcomes measurement in palliative care cannot be overstated. Outcomes measurements are used by PCT leadership to influence the hospital's decision-making on future personnel decisions and other team resource needs. Measurement quantifies information about a palliative care program's impact on clinical, operational, and financial outcomes. Teams that do not collect, analyze, and present data that describe what they do and whom they serve are unlikely to be funded by their executive leadership. According to the Center to Advance Palliative Care (CAPC, 2019), measurement allows programs to:

- Demonstrate value to stakeholders who can serve to justify increased resources and staffing
- Align services with national palliative care quality standards to ensure that programs adhere to best practices

- Manage program operations to describe who is served by the program and how
- Perform continuous quality improvement to monitor the impact of quality improvement efforts over time

The ability to measure outcomes requires strategic planning and alignment, partnerships with analytics and IT to build data collection and extraction processes, and ongoing engagement with the PCT. Outcomes measurement can be a time-consuming challenge that palliative care professionals often loathe—"I just want to take care of my patients!" A significant contributing factor to clinicians' aversion to data management is that few have received adequate training in

BOX 4.12

A TEAM LEADER REFLECTS: JUSTIFYING THE WORTH OF YOUR PCT

When we got started with our team, no one was really tasked with keeping track of our work, so we just sort of jumped in without a plan. Then, we got really busy with patient care, and nobody had time to deal with data. It's a real Catch-22 where you are too busy to collect information because you don't have enough staff but you can't get more staff because you don't have any data. Part of the problem was we weren't sure what we should be tracking or how to get the data without a bunch of extra work. It just got ridiculous—the hospital took away all of our nonbilling staff and we were caught with no way to argue our case. Eventually, we had to stop and regroup. Those of us left standing carved out a little administrative time for me to focus on this. It was kind of painful—a couple of people had to agree to take on even more patients to give me time but we agreed we were in this together.

We had never submitted data to the National Palliative Care Registry—I guess because it seemed like we didn't have enough information to enter. I consulted a mentor who pointed out that perfection can be the enemy of the good and suggested I just submit our staffing data and numbers of referrals (which we did have). Just this little bit plus our staffing numbers gave me some great graphed out benchmarking data that showed how understaffed we were compared to other programs. Also, for three months, we decided to be diligent about keeping track of the referrals we couldn't get to within 24 hours. We used this, plus some data about readmissions that the quality department was already collecting, and some patient stories to describe our value and resource needs. We just got approval for an RN. It's a start. We hope this position allows us to do more with data, so we can continue to build our program.

outcomes measurement or business planning. Additionally, palliative care professionals may not be afforded the time required to plan, implement, and monitor data management processes successfully, even if they understand the importance of these activities (Box 4.12). Palliative care leaders must be provided with training, resources, and time to focus on outcomes measurement.

PEARLS FROM THE FIELD: PROVIDER AND TEAM TAKEAWAYS

Takeaway 1: PCTs might survive poor leadership, but they will not thrive.

Palliative care teams were created to best leverage the expertise of several disciplines to care for seriously ill patients and their families. Without good formal and informal leadership, the best a team can hope for is a group of loosely connected individuals from multiple disciplines who attempt to coordinate patient care. Such models fail to capitalize on the strengths of team-based care and may increase stress, frustration, and burnout. With competent leadership, teams can navigate the complexity of palliative care within the complexity of hospital environments with good outcomes for patients and their families. With great leadership, teams can go beyond the achievements of good outcomes with high team member professional satisfaction through good team relationships and great interdisciplinary problem-solving.

Takeaway 2: The unique structure and purpose of PCTs has exciting implications for team leadership.

PCTs are unlike virtually any other work team. Most individuals in leadership positions manage or oversee other engineers or teachers or accountants. However, in PCTs leaders are tasked with helping professionals from different disciplines come together in order to capitalize on their shared expertise. In high-performing PCTs, member specialization is acknowledged and appreciated for the unique contribution it adds to the strength of the team. In poorly led PCTs, members may find themselves in power struggles with team members from different specialties. In this case, the PCT and the organization may lose good employees who are sick of the politics of the team. Considering the complexity of PCTs, team leaders can improve team functioning by encouraging an environment of leadership at all levels on the team. An environment of leadership stresses the development of all employees, personal accountability, transparency, and intentional communication.

(continued next page)

Takeaway 3: Leadership is a communication skill that can always be honed.

In its simplest form, leadership means to influence. Even when we influence our team to eat lunch together or to tackle conflict in a direct and healthy manner, we are communicating as leaders. However, more often, we think of influence as an obvious formal task as in communicating to encourage someone to share an opinion during a team meeting. The act of leading is communicative by nature. Thus, focusing on and honing communication fundamentals such as immediacy behaviors and relationship development and maintenance is a direct route for enhancing leadership abilities. Leaders may also take time to reflect on the quality of the relationship they share with each individual member and what they can do to ensure that each team member feels valued and appreciated. This may be in the form of tandem goal setting, personalized feedback, or praise. Regardless of the route, team leaders will be most successful when they personalize their communication style to meet the needs of each individual team member and make their decision-making transparent to the team as a whole. Finally, recognizing leadership communication as a skill means that it is something that requires constant attention. Great leaders do not become great because they have figured out communication so well that they no longer have to think about it; they become great through integrating constant vigilance about communication practices into their everyday leadership habits.

References

Back, A. L., Steinhauser, K. E., Kamal, A. H., & Jackson, V. A. (2016). Building resilience for palliative care clinicians: An approach to burnout prevention based on individual skills and workplace factors. *Journal of Pain and Symptom Management, 52*(2), 284–291. doi:10.1016/j.jpainsymman.2016.02.002

Baker, C. R., & Omilion-Hodges, L. M. (2014). The effect of leader-member exchange differentiation within work units on coworker exchange and organizational citizenship behaviors. *Communication Research Reports, 30*, 313–322. doi:10.1080/08824096.2013.837387

Bernerth, J. B., Armenakis, A. A., Feild, H. S., Giles, W. F., & Walker, H. J. (2007). Leader-member social exchange (LMSX): Development and validation of a scale. *Journal of Organizational Behavior, 28*, 979–1003. doi:10.1002/job.443

Center to Advance Palliative Care. (2019, March 4). *Measurement best practices*. Retrieved from https://www.capc.org/toolkits/measurement-best-practices/

Cross, R., Rebele, R., & Grant, A. (2016). Collaborative overload. *Harvard Business Review,* *94*(1–2), 74–79. Retrieved from https://hbr.org/2016/01/collaborative-overload

Cutler, S., Morecroft, C., Carey, P., & Kennedy, T. (2019). Are interprofessional healthcare teams meeting patient expectations? An exploration of the perceptions of patients and informal caregivers. *Journal of Interprofessional Care, 33*(1), 66–75. doi:10.1080/13561 820.2018.1514373

Dahlin, C., Coyne, P., Goldberg, J., & Vaughan, L. (2019). Palliative care leadership. *Journal of Palliative Care, 34,* 21–28. doi:10.1177/0825859718791427

Grant Halvorson, H. (2013, March 14). *The amazing power of 'I Don't' vs. 'I Can't'.* Retrieved from https://www.forbes.com/sites/heidigranthalvorson/2013/03/14/the-amazing-power -of-i-dont-vs-i-cant/#5984d78cd037

Gray, B. (2008). Enhancing transdisciplinary research through collaborative leadership. *American Journal of Preventative Medicine, 35,* S124–S132. doi:10.1016/j.amepre.2008 .03.037

Kelly, S., & Westerman, C. Y. K. (2014). Immediacy as an influence supervisor-subordinate communication. *Communication Research Reports, 31*(3), 252–261. doi:10.1080/08824 096.2014.924335

Lybarger, J. E., Rancer, A. S., & Lin, Y. (2017). Superior-subordinate communication in the workplace: Verbal aggression, nonverbal immediacy, and their joint effects on perceived superior credibility. *Communication Research Reports, 34*(2), 124–133. doi:10.1080/088 24096.2016.1252909

Mehrabian, A. (1981). *Silent messages: Implicit communication of emotions and attitudes.* Belmont, CA: Wadsworth Publishing Company.

Nancarrow, S. A., Booth, A., Ariss, S., Smith, T., Enderby, P., & Roots, A. (2013). Ten principles of good interdisciplinary team work. *Human Resources for Health, 11,* 11–19. doi:10.1186/1478-4491-11-19

Omilion-Hodges, L. M., & Baker, C. R. (2013). Contextualizing LMX within the workgroup: The effects of LMX and justice on relationship quality and resource sharing among peers. *The Leadership Quarterly, 24,* 935–939. doi:10.1177/2329488416687052

Omilion-Hodges, L. M., & Baker, C. R. (2014). Everyday talk and convincing conversations: Utilizing strategic internal communication. *Business Horizons, 57*(3), 435–445. doi:10.1016/j.bushor.2014.02.002

Omilion-Hodges, L. M., & Baker, C. R. (2017). Communicating leader-member relationship quality: The development of leader communication exchange scales to measure relationship building and maintenance through the exchange of communication-based goods. *International Journal of Business Communication, 54*(2), 115–145. doi:10.1177/ 2329488416687052

Payne, M. (2006). Identity politics in multiprofessional teams: Palliative care social work. *Journal of Social Work, 6*(2), 137–150. doi:10.1177/1468017306066741

Sherony, K. M., & Green, S. G. (2002). Coworker exchange: Relationships between coworkers, leader-member exchange, and work attitudes. *Journal of Applied Psychology, 87,* 542–548. doi:10.1037/0021-9010.87.3.542

Stevens, D., & Reifsnyder, J. (2018). Improving team effectiveness: Team health and resilience. *Presentation for Center to Advance Palliative Care.* Retrieved from https://www.capc.org/ events/recorded-webinars/improving-team-effectiveness-team-health-and-resilience/

Turnage, A. K., & Goodboy, A. K. (2016). E-mail and face-to-face organizational dissent as a function of leader-member exchange status. *International Journal of Business Communication, 53*(3), 271–285. doi:10.1177/2329488414525456

Varma, A., & Stroh, L. K. (2001). Different perspectives on selection for international assignments: The impact of LMX and gender. *Cross Cultural Management: An International Journal, 8*(3–4), 85–97. doi:10.1108/13527600110797290

Wayne, S. J., Shore, L. M., & Liden, R. C. (1997). Perceived organizational support and leader- member exchange: A social exchange perspective. *Academy of Management Journal, 40*, 82–111. doi:10.2307/257021

Weick, K. (1995). *Sensemaking in organizations.* Thousand Oaks, CA: Sage.

Weick, K. (2005). Managing the unexpected: Complexity as distributed sensemaking. In R. R. McDaniel & D. J. Dreibe (Eds.), *Uncertain and surprise in complex systems: Question on working with the unexpected* (pp. 51–78). Berlin: Springer-Verlag.

CHAPTER 5

INTERDISCIPLINARY PALLIATIVE CARE TEAM MEETINGS

Introduction

As discussed in Chapter 1, Why We Need to Talk About Teams and Communication in Palliative Care, working in palliative care can be one of the most challenging and simultaneously most rewarding experiences in healthcare delivery due to the focus on providing goal-concordant care (Sanders, Curtis, & Tulsky, 2018). The process of matching the care plan for the patient and family to the patient's own goals and values is complicated by the fact that in the palliative world, providing goal-concordant care is a team effort. In addition to the tremendous amount of emotional labor and clinical expertise required for work in palliative care, communication among team members must be competent, frequent, and consciously maintained to achieve good team outcomes, which lead to better patient/family outcomes. Whether the palliative care team (PCT) is using an interdisciplinary or transdisciplinary model, there will be challenges and opportunities for team communication. Communication is the basis for team coordination, and the most frequently used vehicle for team coordination is the team meeting. Some may think of meetings as the place where productive time goes to die and they would be in good company thinking so. However, professionals in all fields can break the model of the awful meeting with thoughtful planning and an understanding of group communication.

Negative Palliative Care Experience

Nurse Perspective: My team meetings are at best a waste of time and, at worst, dehumanizing. At our weekly meeting, the doctors sit front and center, while the nurses, social workers, and chaplains sit on the outside. The doctors lead the meeting and control the conversation. They focus on what they care about, and they think they are being interdisciplinary if they remember to ask the nurses or social workers for their input. They never ask the chaplains anything at all.

A podcast to accompany this chapter is available with online access of this title. Please see the instructions on the first page of the book for details on how to access and go to Chapter 5.

Positive Palliative Care Experience

Social Worker Perspective: Sometimes, it is hard to make time for our team meetings, but I'm so glad that we do. It really helps me with patient care to be able to talk to everyone else who has interacted with my patients and their families. The team meeting is also our vehicle for making sure that we've covered all the areas (medical, spiritual, social) for the patient and for problem-solving as a group. When I start to feel burnt out, sitting with my team for that hour helps me to recharge even though that time is work. Sometimes the other hospital physicians or administrators make me feel that my job is not as important. But during my team meetings, I'm reminded that I'm valuable because the whole team—doctors, social workers, chaplains, pharmacists, and other nurses—looks to everyone else on the team for input.

Why We Meet

Given the multiple disciplines involved in palliative care, PCTs work best when both the formal and informal meeting structures are well understood by all team members. Frequent formal and informal team meetings can bolster an individual's clinical knowledge while also providing a sense of belonging and a related network of resources (Box 5.1).

BOX 5.1

A RESIDENT REFLECTS: FEELING VALUED DURING TEAM MEETINGS

Tessa is an internal medicine resident completing a rotation with a high-performing transdisciplinary palliative care team.

I don't have to explain myself as much here [on the PCT]. I can make a point, and everyone's like, "Oh, so what you're saying is—" They could finish my sentence for me. My residency has been ICU heavy, and it's not like that in the ICU. On the PCT, they understand what motivates my questions and they have an interest in that motivation.

They also have an interest in discussing and problem-solving. I could make the comment to an ICU doctor and say, "The wife is the decision-maker." And he couldn't care less. Cardiologist is saying "No. No matter what, this is what we are doing," and I remind them that the patient's wife does all the decision-making. And everyone just stares at me. Whereas this team would say, "Right. Well, that's a problem because she's not been coming in here. How are we going to get her to come in?" This team jumps to why I'm pointing that out. It's so much less energy to have that conversation with this team than with my other hospital rotations. I mean, we actually get to have the conversation on the PCT. We are all different specialties, and we get to talk about all the psychosocial aspects of what might be going on plus the biomedical aspects.

For example, through observations and interviews with a high-performing, transdisciplinary PCT at St. Martha's Hospital (pseudonym), Imes and Hester (2014, 2015) found that team members made conscious efforts to create a goal-oriented environment where their values and actions aligned. The authors found that this mindful approach to the coordinated delivery of palliative care resulted in positive organizational, team, and individual outcomes. These benefits largely stem from the fact that all members of this high-performing PCT commit to delivering the highest standard of care possible and they found that to achieve this standard they need to practice high-level interpersonal and group communication. This chapter discusses how to run palliative care meetings that are productive for the team and personally fulfilling for the individuals involved.

Coordination of Goals

PCTs have a number of goals to accomplish. They must attend to the day-to-day medical, psychosocial, and spiritual needs of the patient as well as the needs of the family while also doing future planning for the patient. In interdisciplinary and transdisciplinary teams, members work together to fulfill superordinate goals. Superordinate goals are those that individuals alone cannot satisfy, or satisfy to the extent that the coordinated efforts of a group can (Olsen, Jason, Davidson, & Ferrari, 2009).

In the multidisciplinary model of palliative care, while individual providers—such as physicians, nurses, social workers, pharmacists, or chaplains—provide distinct care and expertise to patients, they can only offer care bound by the parameters of their expertise. However, when these providers join efforts, they are able to offer comprehensive and holistic patient-centered care. Moreover, by working within an interdisciplinary or transdisciplinary team, professionals are also able to connect with others as a means to share and make sense of patient information, grow as professionals, and garner social support from others who work in emotional labor-intensive positions.

PCTs often work best in the transdisciplinary model when the group is able to go beyond the members' usual job descriptions while still recognizing that portions of their roles need particular expertise (e.g., pharmacists are unlikely to know particulars about hospice placement). Transdisciplinary role fluidity also allows for nimble and efficient daily workflow among team members as patient/family needs or staffing issues require. For example, if a team's social worker is out sick or occupied with another patient, a nurse may flex further into psychosocial aspects than usual, turning the work back to the social worker when he or she becomes available or if the patient's needs surpass the nurse's scope of knowledge.

Team Meetings

Meetings are a necessity for high-performing teams. When properly orchestrated, meetings allow teams to coordinate outcomes, deliver top-notch patient care, and often result in the development of trusting professional and personal relationships. Kauffeld and Lehmann-Willenbrock (2012) found that employing an action planning and problem-solving approach to meetings may generate more positive attitudes toward meetings and commitment to achieving group goals.

Advantages and Disadvantages of Team Meetings

Everyone has endured poorly organized and poorly led meetings. However, if done well, meetings can propel interdisciplinary and transdisciplinary teams to heightened levels of patient care because they dedicate time to working toward goal-concordant care. When meetings are organized:

- Vast amounts of information can be conveyed in a short amount of time
- All members work from common, shared expectations
- Members use and react to real-time information
- Problem-solving efficiency can increase as all needed voices and perspectives are in the same room at the same time.

Team meetings build in shared time for members to exchange professionally and sometimes personally (think lunch or coffee breaks). Relatedly, research shows that proximity is an indicator of the development of friendship and a sense of belonging. This interpersonal cohesiveness in groups can help to buffer the factors that lead to burnout on PCTs. Trusting peer and team relationships also promotes more structured, supportive workgroups in addition to spurring member creativity (Omilion-Hodges & Ackerman, 2018). Well-run meetings for high-performing teams can help members to thrive in their profession.

Before developing an interdisciplinary or transdisciplinary team, it is important that members discuss and agree on meeting ground rules. The ground rules should address the frequency and the length of meetings as well as guidelines for how early agendas are issued and protocols for adding to or tabling items. Groups should also

BOX 5.2

DEVIL'S ADVOCATE

While team communication literature often cites the need for a devil's advocate as a constant and rotating member of the team, long-standing groups such as PCTs might find that advice odd. The purpose of a devil's advocate role is to ensure good decision-making by providing a routinized means of dissent. If the team is functioning well, there may not be a need for this as a regular role.

The following are the symptoms that indicate you may need to try a devil's advocate role:

- Some team members regularly hold an informal meeting after the formal meeting to say what they wanted to say during the meeting but felt it would be received as a challenge by other team members.

- Team members find themselves regularly amending the care plans and wondering why the members who knew that information did not share it.

- Team members express "no one listens to me" comments during or outside of meeting times.

All of these symptoms may be the result of the purposeful or accidental silencing of team members. As this type of communication culture can be difficult to change quickly once it is noticed, assigning a devil's advocate for a few meetings may bring the change the team needs. Members will likely find this method annoying, but it will bring attention to the legitimacy of multiple voices on the team.

appoint a timekeeper for each meeting and consider assigning a rotating devil's advocate role. These group and meeting roles allow teams to judiciously address task demands while remaining cognizant of relational dynamics. For example, if each group member takes a turn assuming the role of the devil's advocate, then it allows the group to consider potential consequences while separating the issue from the individual issuing them (Box 5.2). By rotating through the role of the devil's advocate, individual members are empowered to speak up and help the group to consider possible consequences or alternatives of the predominant or prevailing point of view. Relatedly, assigning group members to play the role of the timekeeper helps to keep the group on task while respecting all members' time.

Just like the discussion of best practices and the challenges of team leaders in Chapter 3, Formation and Maintenance of High-Performing Palliative Care Teams, team meetings have similar challenges. The three challenges discussed here are balancing task and relationship agendas, time commitment, and handling dissent in groups.

Task and Relationship Agendas

Balancing task and relationship communication agendas is an issue in all forms of interpersonal communication. In the workplace, that balance may tip toward task agendas due to the perception that the task is the purpose of the group. However, PCTs become high-performing through interpersonal cohesiveness. While too much cohesiveness can result in groupthink, groups can thrive with enough cohesiveness to make members feel valued and important. Practice and mindfulness can keep a group from sliding from positive cohesion into groupthink (Box 5.3).

BOX 5.3

GROUPTHINK

High levels of cohesion are one element of high-performing teams. However, Janis (1982) noted close-knit teams sometimes became high-cohesion/poor decision-making teams when "members striving for unanimity override their motivation to realistically appraise alternative courses of action." Kaba et al. (2016) indicate that medical teams are not immune to poor decision making due to groupthink. Janis identified the following factors as indicators that groupthink was endangering high-quality decision-making:

- Collective rationalization
- Self-censorship
- Direct pressure on dissenters
- Self-appointment mind guards

A study of interdisciplinary education using simulations found both medical and nursing students were likely to bend to the pressure of group conformity when discussing vital signs. However, nursing students were "significantly more likely to conform to the opinion of medical students than vice versa" (Kaba & Beran, 2016). Should such habits carry over into interdisciplinary palliative care teams, high-quality group decision-making would be endangered.

Handling Dissent

While many are uncomfortable with conflict, it is ubiquitous in groups. As discussed in Chapter 3, Formation and Maintenance of High-Performing Palliative

Care Teams, when done well, conflict is productive and leads to higher quality group decisions. Jehn (1995) distinguished three types of group conflicts: task, relationship, and process. Of the three types, relationship conflict is usually seen as the least functional as it makes the conflict personal. However, Garner and Iba (2017) found that task and process dissent can also influence the group as "group members were likely to ostracize an idea dissenter and potentially to look upon a process dissenter as a leader" (p. 355). An understanding of the ways dissenters are viewed and sometimes silenced is particularly important in team meetings. While the "show of hands" means of making a decision works for some groups, PCTs are making decisions about the quality of a person's life and death, a family's experience, and providers' actions. Thus, working to create consensus, as discussed in Chapter 3, Formation and Maintenance of High-Performing Palliative Care Teams, has the greatest likelihood of creating a high-quality decision for the team as well as for patients and families.

One difficulty in team meetings can be distinguishing dissent from obstruction. Dissent is a different perspective that complicates decision-making but ultimately adds important information to the process, whereas the purpose of obstruction is stopping a decision-making process or ensuring that nothing challenges the status quo. Obstructors are sometimes identified as *disruptors*. Although disruptors are often perceived as those working to disrupt the status quo, in this case the disruptors are upholding the status quo by disrupting any attempt to change the way decisions are made. Shapiro and Nadelman (2014) offer this perspective on dealing with disruptors who are also high in the power hierarchy, saying, "Disruptors tend to see themselves as staunch patient advocates and those who do not stand with them as people who are not as committed to patient care as they [are]" (p. 79). These authors also point out that this obstructionist method has likely worked in the obstructor's favor in the past and so they continue with the behavior. The obstructor's organizational status may make it difficult to see how to work with them, as a well-functioning group does welcome dissent and the disruptors may cloak their desire not to change as dissent. Disruptive communication behaviors such as these are bad for group decision-making and they can also have negative repercussions on patient safety outcomes (The Joint Commission [TJC], 2008). Disruptors may be weeded out through the group-forming process (discussed in Chapter 3, Formation and Maintenance of High-Performing Palliative Care Teams). If they are not, appeals to the group's goals of maximizing effective and compassionate care for seriously ill patients and their families may help disruptors to see that they are not alone—everyone is committed to patient and family care. Should this appeal not suffice, team leaders and Human Resources may need to work with this team member on coaching for proactive team communication behaviors.

Time Commitment

Interdisciplinary and transdisciplinary teams offer a wonderful opportunity for goal-concordant care for patients and a context in which to thrive for team members. However, these types of teams do take more time, particularly in the formation stages, to achieve this group norm. Once the team is established, if mindful communication is left out because "we did that to get started and now we know what we are doing," the group can regress from being effective and efficient to burned out and angry. Building time into the group formation and maintenance processes to practice and critique group communication is vital. St. Martha's PCT negotiated time for team building and process development when they agreed to form a new team. As the years have passed, especially during times of under-staffing or high patient care demands, they remind one another to make time for consciously tending to team communication. At various times since the PCT's formation, they have tried to save time by having fewer meetings. However, they discovered that failure to make time for team building, information sharing, process improvement, and grief work hurts them in the long run. One PCT nurse told us, "If you don't tend the garden, you'll have nothing to harvest." If your team is already functioning, or if you are unable to negotiate the time prior to starting your team, building time into your weekly meetings at the beginning can create the space for these processes. Additionally, carving out time for an annual team retreat can help your group to cover a lot of communicative ground in a shorter amount of time.

Start as You Mean to Go On: Setting Up the Structure and Norms for Successful Team Meetings

Work teams have several different types of meetings (Table 5.1). Meetings that usually involve the entire PCT include patient coordination meetings and administrative coordination meetings. Of the two types, patient coordination meetings are frequent and often a part of the set daily schedule. Administrative coordination meetings are weekly/bimonthly/monthly and include programmatic issues that relate to the larger organization under which the PCT functions. These meetings may also have professional development components. Some teams also schedule a yearly retreat day for team building and professional development.

TABLE 5.1 **Meeting Types**

TYPES	PURPOSE	ATTENDEES	FREQUENCY
Examples of Formal Meetings			
Rounds (around the table or mobile)	• Start the day • Regroup • Primary purpose: Coordinate patient care • Note problem patterns—to be addressed at team meetings	Everyone on service that day	Daily

Team meetings	• Broader topics for PCTs
	  • How are we handling ____?
	  • What is the latest research on ____?
	• Time for more intentional team communication than hallway conversations
		Everyone (those off service are encouraged to attend)	Weekly or Monthly

Retreats	• Emotional care of the team as a group • Broader topic focus than in team meetings (e.g., compassion fatigue) • Reconnect as a full team	Everyone	Annually
Examples of Informal Meetings			
Lunch	• Time to eat • Work and personal discussions mix • Decompress with other ingroup members	Anyone who can and wants to attend	Daily

(continued)

TABLE 5.1 **Meeting Types** (*continued*)

TYPES	PURPOSE	ATTENDEES	FREQUENCY
Happy hour	• Time to enjoy one another's company • Decompress outside the hospital environment	Anyone who can and wants to attend	Monthly
Holiday party	• Celebrate by expressing the value of the team and its members • Social connections • Reconnect as a full team	Everyone	Annually

Because meetings are such an omnipresent part of work life, many people approach them as an obligation whose form, format, and function are predetermined by the fact that it is a meeting. Assumptions about meetings include the following:

- There will be an agenda.
- People will pay varying amounts of attention.
- Some work will get done, but lots will not.
- Most people would rather be somewhere else.

Continuing to conduct meetings without a thoughtful structure, predetermined norms, and negotiated group roles can add to the stress and frustration of team members. As healthcare and palliative care, in particular, are already stress-laden jobs, learning to do meetings better is an investment in personnel and patients. Teams that begin their process by talking about how they want to communicate during meetings are most likely to achieve favorable meeting attitudes, and those favorable attitudes are predictive of high-performing teams (O'Neill & Allen, 2012).

This conscious attention to communication is also called mindful communication. Mindful communication brings two concepts together into a single practice: adaptive and reflexive communication with an emphasis on remaining present and aware. While the concept is easy to grasp, it is an active process that requires practice for individuals to learn how to stay focused and attentive to situational factors such as audience, context, and goals of communicative exchanges. When practiced in the clinical setting, mindful communication has been linked with enhanced patient care and decreases in provider burnout (Anthony & Vidal, 2010; Beckman et al., 2012). Omilion-Hodges and Swords (2016) found four key mindful communication practices commonly employed by palliative care providers:

1. Know your audience
2. Ask questions
3. Discard scripts
4. Recognize your role

While these practices will be discussed more thoroughly in Chapter 6, Occupational Culture: Understanding the Role and Stigma of Palliative Care, applying the concept of mindful communication to team, patient, and family meetings will help palliative care professionals to be more successful in collaborating effectively with peers and in communicating difficult information to patients and families.

Part of mindful communication includes thinking through the logistics of how groups function well and enculturating these best practices into your daily group process. Groups might assign specific tasks for team members, including:

- someone who looks up and reports clinical information,
- someone who ensures complete and accurate documentation,
- someone who keeps time, and
- someone who tracks and summarizes the daily assignments at the end of the meeting.

If these individual tasks are defined and valued by the team as a whole, it becomes possible to complete or correct documentation deficiencies, to ensure that all disciplines are heard, and to ensure that the meeting ends on time. Responsibility for each task may be rotating, or the team might identify individuals' strengths that allow them to excel at specific roles. A benefit of rotating responsibility for these tasks is that all members have the chance to consider the challenges and benefits associated with each while also taking more ownership in the outcome of the meeting and of the team.

The Importance of Formal Team Meetings

PCTs may have regularly scheduled meetings for the purpose of announcements, continuing education, logistical planning, acknowledging the deaths of patients, and complying with the needs of the larger organization in which they are embedded. The structure of these meetings is often similar to those in many other fields. There is likely to be an agenda, the agenda may be upended if a more pressing issue is at hand, and some members might not attend if other work needs are deemed to be more important. When PCTs have high-frequency interactions and busy patient loads, some may perceive that these more traditional meetings are too time-consuming and should be dropped. However, this type of meeting does allow for team coordination and team education, and keeping it in the schedule is encouraged (Box 5.4).

BOX 5.4

PROVIDER REFLECTIONS: "DO WE REALLY NEED THIS MEETING?"
Our team went through a particularly brutal period of time when we were short staffed and patient volume was high. All of us were working 10 to 12 hours a day just to get through our patient care. Weekly team meetings started to feel like an annoyance and a luxury of the past when we could find time to come together. Weeks went by where we didn't meet at all or, if we did, only a few people would come—and they would be antsy to get back out to the floor. As time went on, some of the structures we had in place, like taking time to teach each other things, paying attention to performance improvement, and acknowledging patient deaths, fell away.

A few times, people got annoyed that they didn't know something was happening in the hospital or with the team, but there was never any opportunity or forum to just be together and talk through it. We found a way to carve out a retreat day by bringing in prn (as needed) staff. In addition to finally having a chance to work through our stress and tend to self-care, the whole team was able to acknowledge that our team meetings were valuable and necessary. Some people noticed that changes in workflow or documentation were needed to meet patient needs, but without the team meeting, it wasn't possible to develop new processes. Others noticed that we had begun to lose our much valued "culture of learning" by never taking time to review new articles. The good news was, prior to this really hard time, we had solidified our way of doing things enough that we had a structure to return to. We did make some adjustments to make meetings more productive and meaningful like putting time limits on the agenda and moving the start time 30 minutes later, but mostly, we just recommitted to the practice. We learned that yes, we really did need this meeting for our team to be a high-performing group that provided excellent patient care and helped one another to avoid burnout.

While most healthcare professionals partake in a variety of meetings, PCTs engage in patient coordination meetings daily. These meetings are different than most other types of meetings in a variety of ways, but most distinct is the level of complexity that patient coordination meetings require in terms of integration of various participants and the various goals of each participant. The next section focuses on how to engage in productive patient coordination meetings.

Patient Coordination Meetings or "Rounds"

The purpose of patient coordination meetings is to coordinate goal-concordant patient care among team members with different areas of expertise and different levels of experience with the individual patients and families on the team's census. Because excellent patient care is the primary purpose of the healthcare team, PCTs who hold frequent, regularly scheduled patient coordination meetings are most likely to become high-performing teams. Whenever possible, the discussions about team meeting communication should happen as a part of team formation. However, the reality is that many PCTs have already formed and would like to communicate better. The list of communication considerations for meetings presented in Exhibit 5.1 can be addressed during team formation or at any point when the PCT decides, through experience, that adjustments should be made to improve communication.

EXHIBIT 5.1

WHO'S ON FIRST AND WHAT'S ON SECOND? UNPACKING TEAM COMMUNICATION CONSIDERATIONS

Clear communication is not always easy, and it becomes even more challenging in high-stressed situations such as palliative care. However, taking the time to discuss some of the following considerations will help to minimize misunderstandings so your time can actually be spent working (gasp!) instead of trying to figure out who is taking minutes, who is writing the agenda, and so on.

Who? Personnel-related questions

- Who will be present?
  - Some teams have a core team who work full time on the PCT with other members who work part-time or who work on one week, off the next.
  - Some teams may be moving between multiple hospitals within the same system.

How? Administrative nuts and bolts

- How often should we meet?
- How long should the meeting be?
- How can we run the meeting so we are thorough, but also efficient?
- How will we act during the meeting?
- Can members be on phones/devices? If so, under what circumstances?
- Are we all business or will we also have fun? If we allow for jokes/commentary, how will we make enough room to enjoy one another while still being efficient with our time?
- How will we handle documentation during the meeting?

What? Setting boundary conditions and communication behavior expectations

- How will we address conflict?
- Should all conflict be addressed the same way?
- Should different opinions about patient care be addressed upfront and during the meeting? If not then, when?
- Should personal differences about communication styles and/or perceived interpersonal conflict between team members be handled outside of the patient coordination time?
- What work circumstances (if any) should be prioritized above the attendance of this meeting?

Example: *Day-to-day patient coordination*—St. Martha's PCT, the high-performing exemplar studied by Imes and Hester, begins each day with 45–60 minutes of morning rounds. These are table rounds—conducted in a conference room with access to the electronic medical record (patient chart)—rather than hospital rounds that are face-to-face with the patient. The purpose of this PCT's morning rounds is coordination of care, and daily table rounds have been a part of the team process since the team formation. Table rounds allow everyone to be on the same page for that day as well as catch up with any patient changes or conversations with patients or families that occurred since the previous day. Table rounds can be structured in a way that embodies mindful communication at work (Exhibit 5.1). In addition to serving the purpose of patient coordination, the table rounds routine is a gateway for becoming focused and present at work (Box 5.5).

BOX 5.5

FUNCTIONS OF TABLE ROUNDS AT ST. MARTHA'S

1. Efficiently engage the full interdisciplinary team in clinical recommendations for medication choices, communication strategies, and so on
2. Plan the day:
   - Determine which team members need to see each patient
   - Identify specific tasks or unmet patient needs
   - Assign new patients
3. Ensure that documentation requirements are completed.

As referral volume grows, it may not be practical to expand the length of the meeting time. In order to maintain full team engagement, the meeting agenda must be clear, and each PCT member should feel invited to share relevant and timely information for each patient. Team members may be assigned specific tasks during this meeting. One team member may be tasked with facilitating the meeting—reviewing and communicating clinical information from the electronic health record, tracking team assignments, and ensuring all disciplines have an opportunity to weigh in. Another team member may be tasked with quality assurance and identifying and communicating deficits in required documentation. It can be helpful to designate one team member to watch the clock. While moments of levity are encouraged to keep the team engaged and to lighten spirits, the team should snap back to focus without complaint when a time constraint is noted. At the end of the meeting, the meeting facilitator should review the entire patient list—each patient name is read aloud along with the names of the team members who are responsible for care that day. This practice encourages accountability and helps identify lopsided assignments that may require some redistribution of responsibility. In high-performing teams, members are able to let one another know when they feel someone has "flexed" into an area they have already covered. In teams with low-function communication, such a statement could be face-threatening and seen as inappropriate. In the following example, however, the corrective communication functions to allow the team to coordinate and move on with ease:

Dianne (APRN): *So I don't know what to do. I mean, I'll talk to his nurse, too, because I know with delirium, if it clears, you can have more awareness of your pain. It looked like, overnight, he actually didn't get that much hydromorphone.*

Catie (APRN):   [reading chart] *Pain looks a little better. Wait. I just noticed. Do we have the right next of kin information in here?*

Linnea (RN):   *Hey. Stay in your lane, Catie.* [Laughs] *I'm responsible for that.*

As mentioned previously, rotating roles during the meetings is a pragmatic way to enhance accountability. For example, by taking turns being the time keeper, it becomes easier to recognize the stress that side chatter places on meeting productivity and on the individual who is charged with keeping the group on task. Thus, these roles, while transitory, provide team members with a sense of leadership and mutual respect within the group. Additionally, members who feel empowered to share their opinions or who are looking for structure, expertise, or guidance are more committed to long-term group and organizational successes (Harrison & Killion, 2007).

Another approach is to identify individual team member's strengths and leverage those strengths by assigning a specific role with the explicit agreement by the rest of the team (Box 5.6). For example, if one person tends to be particularly detail oriented, that team member might be assigned the task of ensuring complete and accurate documentation during the meeting. This ensures team-identified quality measures, such as dyspnea screening and comprehensive pain assessment, are not neglected. When everyone has a common understanding of the expectations and agrees that this team member has been empowered to identify documentation deficiencies (either publicly, during the meeting, or privately, after the meeting), the PCT can remain accountable to regulatory requirements in an ongoing manner. Team leaders can further empower members by stressing the importance of meeting roles and leading a conversation about what can and will likely happen if someone is not charged with critical tasks.

BOX 5.6

PROVIDER REFLECTIONS: THE RIGHT PERSON FOR THE JOB

Our PCT has one clinician who likes to just get out there and do. She gets antsy during meetings if she's not actively engaged in whatever is being talked about and feels frustrated when meetings drag on. During a recent team meeting, we decided to leverage her strengths by moving her into the role of "running rounds" (looking up and reporting clinical information). For each patient discussed, she is able to quickly process relevant patient information and ensure that all disciplines have the chance to speak. It was a revelation to find a solution that simultaneously keeps her engaged and makes our meeting more efficient. Ending on time with all the information we need to tackle the day is like being gifted an extra 15 to 30 minutes, and everybody is happier.

The Importance of Informal Meetings

In the realm of informal meetings, breaks such as lunch can also offer interdisciplinary teams an opportunity to check in on professional and personal concerns. Returning to St. Martha's PCT, core members try to eat lunch together as often as possible rather than eating alone at their desks. While this "meeting" is much less formal than morning rounds, it provides the team brief, unstructured time to talk about work or share personal information. Additionally, while there is no associated agenda, a fair amount of professional processing may take place over a meal. Moreover, this informal time together not only helps to onboard and socialize new members, but it also often provides a much-needed reprieve from the stressors of clinical care. Thus, the fluidity that results from the daily lunch break also reiterates the goals shared by members of the team and a commitment to the delivery of outstanding palliative care. This strategy for collaborative work, of course, requires physical accommodations for gathering—a resource request that should be prioritized whenever possible. Informal gathering over lunch does mean that team members rarely get a break from one another. Ideas about balancing high-frequency contact with team members' need for physical and emotional space from one another are addressed in Chapter 7, Self-Care and Team Care in Emotional Labor-Intensive Positions.

In high-performing interdisciplinary teams, the consistent and direct use of communication is the preferred route for addressing patient- and personnel-related concerns. That direct communication can take place face-to-face or via texting. The use of cellphones by PCTs is consistent with studies of various medical specialties (Wyber, Khashram, Donnell, & Meyer-Rochow, 2013) indicating that medical providers report using their personal cell phones as a means to share results, logistics, and management of clinical cases as well as to make social arrangements. Teams who are mindful of their interactions include consideration of the best channel (i.e., face-to-face, email, texting) for communicating different types of information.

Virtual Versus Face-to-Face Teamwork

It is increasingly easier to collaborate across geographic boundaries. Given the ubiquity of cell phones in the workplace, PCT members communicate via text messages in order to exchange information, seek another opinion, or offer social support in real time. Many professionals, especially in fast-paced medical settings, prefer virtual communication such as the use of text messages as a means to engage with team members. Convenience, reliability, less intrusion, and face-saving responses were all cited as reasons why employing technology or communicating virtually was preferred (Wyber et al., 2013). While texting may be a preferred means of interacting, healthcare organizations are working to walk the line between technology that speeds professional communication while simultaneously protecting patient privacy (see Box 5.7).

While virtual or non–face-to-face communication does offer some clear benefits, it should not comprise the majority of team interaction, as communication researchers have found that physical proximity offers additional advantages for team cohesion and problem-solving. In fact, overreliance on remote means of

BOX 5.7

TO TEXT OR NOT TO TEXT? THAT IS THE HIPAA QUESTION

With the ubiquity of smartphones, it is no surprise that healthcare professionals rely on their devices for several professional reasons. It is also no surprise that healthcare organizations seem to be constantly playing catchup with new technology implementations. This communication channel sits at the nexus of competing goals in healthcare: fast connection of healthcare professionals for the purpose of providing good care and protection of patient privacy. Teams and organizations have several considerations for utilizing texting and encrypted messaging.

1. Patient care

   Patient care is a tricky area for the use of messaging. While The Joint Commission's 2016 directive banned the use of texting for patient care orders, there are many other areas of patient care that must also be protected. Most teams use encrypted messaging to discuss patients or seek clarification on orders. Healthcare systems may prefer that providers use the electronic medical record peer-to-peer functions for these discussions; however, in the fast-paced world of hospital work, providers are more likely to use the messaging technologies available on their phones.

2. Coordinating logistics

   Texting has become the virtual assistant of our days. It facilitates finding times to meet, figuring out who said they would do what, and informing colleagues that someone will be late, among many other functions. As these types of communication do not contain sensitive information, no encrypted programs are necessary.

3. Coordination of relational meaning

   As texting does not contain nonverbal cues, it can often be the cause of misunderstandings between people. Conversely, it can also be used to clear up misunderstandings. For example, one morning a PCT nurse had an encounter with a team physician that left her confused about the relational meaning of the conversation. She perceived that the physician was annoyed with her based on her read of his nonverbal communication but she did not believe she had done anything that merited a negative response from the physician team member. As a means to help make sense of the interaction, the nurse texted a fellow team member who was able to clarify what the physician meant, thereby alleviating the miscommunication and related relationship uncertainty.

4. Team bonding

The group text serves to relay information to others and also to share jokes, frustrations, or funny things that happen during the day. While this is on the personal end of the spectrum, it still has the professional purpose of an ongoing creation of the team bond.

interacting can impact both team relationships and problem-solving. Meeting requisite variety, or the amount of variability in problem-solving that matches the level of complexity of the problem, requires information-rich channel sources, as they carry the most contextual clues to interpreting meaning. Weick (2001) explains "information richness declines as people move away from face to face interaction ... too much richness introduces the inefficiencies of over complication, too little media richness introduces the inaccuracy of oversimplification" (p. 333). When face-to-face meetings are well led, the inefficiencies can be avoided. However, if team members are unaware of the contextual cues that they are missing in the least information-rich channels such as texting, the inaccuracies may be hard to catch. PCTs may use administrative meetings or yearly retreats as a time to discuss when texting is being used productively or when team members may be "hiding" behind their phones, coming to agreement when communication would be improved upon by calling one another or interacting face-to-face.

Sias, Pedersen, Gallagher, and Kopaneva (2012) found that while personality and opportunities to work together remain important facets in the development of workplace friendships, physical proximity ceased to be a factor in their respondents' abilities to initiate workplace friendships. This indicates that high-performing teams whose function is at least partially linked to members liking one another need not rely on constant physical presence to initiate or maintain feelings of collegiality and bondedness. Teams should strive for balance, however, as one of the structural threats to team health is "minimal team contact" (Stevens & Reifsnyder, 2018, p. 11).

Returning to the exemplar transdisciplinary St. Martha's PCT, members make a concerted effort to maintain communication. Through the integration of formal meetings, such as morning table rounds, and informal meetings, such as sharing lunch, the members create a multitude of opportunities to share and process clinical information. Additionally, members do not wait for these face-to-face meetings to consider new information—rather they engage in regular hallway and virtual conversations when confronted with new, ambiguous, or otherwise confusing news. In this sense, communication in formal and informal team meetings becomes the primary vehicle for coordinating goals and delivering first-rate care.

Family Meetings

Meetings with the families of patients is also a type of team meeting for a PCT. The PCT, along with other providers involved with a patient's care, should meet prior to the family meeting to determine the agenda and communication roles (i.e., which team member addresses what issues). Ideally, the healthcare team gets on "the same page" before meeting with a family. This does not imply that everyone must be in agreement about the recommendations for care. However, differences in opinion should not be a surprise during the family meeting. A brief pre-meeting before the family meeting allows divergent opinions to be considered ahead of time so families may receive nuanced and thoughtful information to help guide them through the complexity of a situation, even when facing uncertainty and disagreement. The excerpt (Exhibit 5.2) from morning rounds at a PCT illustrates the struggle when the medical team believes they know what is best for a patient and the family disagrees. As the chaplain says, sometimes it is best to walk with the family and just make sure they are also hearing what the medical team is saying.

EXHIBIT 5.2

A CONVERSATION AT MORNING TABLE ROUNDS LEADS TO RECOMMENDING A FAMILY MEETING

APRN: Okay, let's start with Susan.

Social worker: I followed up with Dr. H yesterday because it seems like folks are sort of avoiding talking to her family at this point. Early on, they were talking about "Well, maybe hospice," but I really talked them down from that because that just wasn't where the family was at. Pushing hospice when the oncologist told her she might still be able to get chemo...it just didn't make sense to her. Things might be changing, though.

APRN: How's her pain been, Lauren?

RN: It seemed better yesterday, but she's kind of lethargic, like, she can't maintain a conversation, but I don't necessarily think that it's because of her morphine PCA. She's just getting weaker.

MD: How are her kidneys doing?

Pharmacist: Yeah, I was just looking at that. Her renal function is worse. Maybe we should consider switching opioids. I can talk to Dr. H about that.

APRN:	How are her husband and sister, Patty, doing these days? I've not seen them. Ramona, you've been in it for the long haul with them...
Chaplain:	You know, I know Patty pretty well now, and I think everyone's getting the wrong idea. They think that she doesn't understand what's happening, but that's not the case. She's hearing what the doctor is saying, but she has a very strong faith belief that Susan's gonna get up and walk outta here, and you know, telling her that her faith is wrong is not gonna help. I don't think it's likely she'll get better, but I think they discount her too quickly as just being an overzealous religious freak—*[laughs]*—you know, and she's not. She just truly feels like God has told her that Susan's gonna get up and walk outta here. So, until, I guess, she and God have a different conversation, I'm just gonna walk alongside and make sure that she is also hearing what the medical team is saying.
APRN:	So, Kathy, you'll talk with Dr. H about switching opioids? And then we need to reach out to Patty about a meeting. Ramona, do you want to see Susan today?
Chaplain:	Yeah, that would be lovely, and I'll see if Patty would be open to meeting with the team to talk about how things are going.

Teams need to devote special attention to their preparations for family meetings. While most guides focus on conducting the meeting itself, Hudson, Quinn, O'Hanlon, and Aranda (2008) include a section on preparing for the meeting:

- Plan time to discuss the family meeting either with the full team or only with the subset of the team who will meet with the family.
- Determine when a family meeting should be offered if the family has not requested one.
- Determine which family members should be invited.
- Identify "the most appropriately skilled person from the team to convene [and lead] the meeting" (p. 7).

Experienced members of PCTs likely learned to run family meetings as a part of on-the-job training. However, due to the growing emphasis on the need for palliative care providers, elements of palliative care practice including conducting family meetings are now reflected in newer medical education practices. Although the study by Hudson et al. (2008) found that "formal training in conducting family meetings does not occur as part of general training" (p. 5), a decade later, such training is beginning. Hagiwara et al. (2018) at the University of Texas Health Science Center at San Antonio tested and refined a Family Meeting Assessment Tool (FMAT), which assesses nine domains of conducting family meetings including general communication skills and cultural, spiritual, and team issues among others. This tool is intended for use with fourth-year medical students (M4s) for formative skill assessments. The domains covered in the FMAT may also prove useful to PCTs in their discussions on professional development and leading family meetings.

A "road map" often used by PCTs for conducting family meetings is detailed by Back, Arnold, and Tulsky (2009) in their book *Mastering Communication with Seriously Ill Patients*. Their eight-step road map elaborates on the SPIKES model for sharing bad news proposed by Ballie et al.—**S**et up, **P**erception, **I**nvitation, **K**nowledge, **E**motions, **S**ummary (Baile et al., 2000). Back et al. add "exploring the patients' values and how they should influence decision-making" (2009, p. 87) as well as preparing to negotiate patient care goals. It is important to remember that these road maps are just maps—and not scripts. Every family has their own story, and the PCT members help guide them to tell that story and find their way through their decision-making. As one palliative care professional says,

> We don't go into these consults with a script. My rule is no script, new people, new story. Every person demands a fresh take and our time is asking questions, getting to know them, and helping to continue and finalize their story as they intend (Omilion-Hodges & Swords, 2017, p. 1279).

One of the unique aspects of PCTs is an often misunderstood element of their practice. As mentioned in other chapters, many people and healthcare providers still believe that palliative care only begins to work with patients and families when a terminal diagnosis occurs and the patient chooses hospice care. In those cases, the PCT may be newly introduced to the patient and family and will know them only for the short time until the patient dies. While that is one of the situations in which PCTs may operate, palliative care referrals can occur any time a patient has a serious illness. Therefore, it is possible that the PCT knows the patient and family quite well when the time comes to make difficult decisions on behalf of the patient. Exhibit 5.3 serves as an exemplar of just how much more a PCT might know about a family than an outside observer. This depth of knowledge along with meeting preparation for the PCT assist the team in helping three sisters make decisions about their mother's care placement.

EXHIBIT 5.3

MINI CASE STUDY: FAMILY CONFERENCES AND THE IMPORTANCE OF PCT INVOLVEMENT OVER TIME

An example of what an observant outsider misses when watching a family conference.

Palliative team members present: APRN, social worker, and chaplain

Patient: 78-year-old woman, in nursing home with advancing dementia. She no longer meets criteria for acute rehab facility placement as she has becoming less interested in food and not participating with OT/PT. The care level and insurance coverage is consistent with placement at one of two long-term care facilities in the area. Her daughters are not in agreement on which facility to choose.

What the researcher observed: Three sisters, aged 45, 47, and 55 years of age, seated near each other in arm chairs in the family meeting room. The youngest and middle daughters lean slightly toward one another and away from the eldest. The youngest daughter seems the most invested in the meeting and decision-making—she sits upright and leans toward the nurse who is the first member of the team to speak. This daughter speaks about her mother's condition and preferences in an authoritative tone and frequently looks for confirmation from middle sister. Both women believe placement A is best for their mother.

The eldest sister sits to the side, and her body curled in on itself in her chair. She orients her body toward her sisters but turns her face away from them and does not look up or give much indication that she has an opinion. Her facial expressions and constantly tearing eyes show that this is a hard conversation for her.

What the observer concluded: Choosing placement A seems simple. The youngest sister appears to know the most about her mother's desire for her care plan, and the middle sister is prepared to support the plan and her sister. The eldest sister is probably sad about her mother's condition and is unlikely to make an effort to be involved in this decision.

What the PCT knows: The eldest sister has been the primary caregiver of the mother for a number of years. This is the first family meeting the youngest and middle sisters have attended. While their choice is for placement A, the eldest prefers placement B because it is closer to her home and will increase the likelihood that she, the older sister, will be able to visit daily. The middle and younger sisters think placement A looks like a nicer facility, but the eldest sister has already confirmed in previous meetings with the PCT that placement B is equally as good of a match for taking care of their mother. The eldest has been annoyed with her sisters' lack of investment in the care decisions for their mother to this point. Now that they have decided to be involved, she is hurt by their advocacy of a different placement and saddened because she sees herself outvoted by her sisters who are unlikely to visit their mother frequently no matter where she is placed.

What the PCT does: The team allows the younger and middle sisters to state their preferences and ask questions of the team. Then the team skillfully draws out the eldest sister's concerns and preferences. When the meeting ends, there is no decision but concrete plans to gather information that addresses the questions and concerns of all three women.

PEARLS FROM THE FIELD: PROVIDER AND TEAM TAKEAWAYS

Maintaining high-performing interdisciplinary or transdisciplinary teams requires ongoing attention to structure and process. One way to maintain a high-performing PCT is through frequent and focused formal and informal meetings. Three key takeaways are discussed in the following.

Takeaway 1: Becoming a high-performing interdisciplinary or transdisciplinary team takes time and mindful processing.

Interprofessional communication is part and parcel of transdisciplinary teams and working within larger, interconnected medical systems. Researchers have long (Frank, 1961) reiterated the challenges that emerge when specialists talk across discipline boundaries. The challenges are not necessarily born out of ill will, but rather because individuals tend to operate from their own mental maps or conceptual frameworks that guide the assumptions, decisions, recommendations, and opinions offered. Thus, if a grouping of various medical professionals is operating from their own mental map, then it is of little surprise why medical errors are common, interdisciplinary teams tend to retreat back to silos, and why members may have challenges valuing other team members' contributions.

Integrating routine and well-orchestrated formal meetings can help move a group of individuals to a high-performing transdisciplinary team. Through the process of setting and working toward coordinated goals, members will need to share information and engage in collective sensemaking. These tasks are achieved through communication, which can occur in face-to-face and mediated settings. Use of technology such as texts and messenger apps allows the exchange of information and processing to take place in real time. This can be

(continued next page)

essential for the delivery of new patient information, or, as was seen in the case of members of the St. Martha's PCT, to address confusion in an exchange among colleagues. Additionally, the use of mediated channels allows team members to continue to work toward coordinated goals without having to wait or linger on various issues before the next scheduled formal face-to-face. While there are a number of benefits of mediated and virtual communication, it is important to remember that face-to-face encounters can facilitate quicker understanding and lead to the development of friendships.

Takeaway 2: Many hands make for a lighter load. When done well, meetings can spur productivity and ease individual workloads.

When done without clear intentions or established ground rules (e.g., time limitations, expectations for communicative behavior), meetings can quickly go awry. Unfortunately, the unstructured and unproductive meeting is so commonplace that virtually everyone can relate to the feelings of annoyance that may arise even at the word *meeting* because meetings can result in a lot of talk and little to no action. However, with planning, shared expectations, and rotating group roles, well-orchestrated meetings can streamline practitioners' workloads.

Takeaway 3: Well-executed meetings enhance team identity.

Meetings can be terrific catalysts for helping to shape a shared team identity, where members are able to identify shared characteristics to begin to answer the "who are we?" question. Meetings are influential in molding identity because of the amount of time members spend together, the shared opinions that lead to collective decisions for patient-concordant care, and the ability of members to support each other in terms of sharing information and knowledge, and many times, compassion and empathy.

References

Anthony, M. K., & Vidal, K. (2010). Mindful communication: A novel approach to improving delegation and increasing patient safety. *Online Journal of Issues in Nursing, 15*(2), Manuscript 2. doi:10.3912/OJIN Vol15No2Man02

Back, A., Arnold, R., & Tulsky, J. (2009). *Mastering communication with seriously ill patients: Balancing honesty with empathy and hope.* New York: Cambridge Press.

Baile, W. F., Buckman, R., Lenzi, R., Glober, G., Beale, E. A., & Kudelka, A. P. (2000). SPIKES—A six-step protocol for delivering bad news: Application to the patient with cancer. *The Oncologist, 5,* 302–311. doi:10.1634/theoncologist.5-4-302

Beckman, H. B., Wendland, M., Mooney, C., Krasner, M. S., Quill, T. E., Suchman, A. L., & Epstein, R. M. (2012). The impact of a program in mindful communication on primary care physicians. *Academic Medicine, 87,* 815–819. doi:10.1097/ACM.0b013 e318253d3b2

Frank, L. K. (1961). Interprofessional communication. *American Journal of Public Health and the Nations Health, 51*(12), 1798–1804. doi:10.2105/AJPH.51.12.1798

Garner, J. T., & Iba, D. L. (2017). Why are you saying that? Increases in gaze duration as responses to group member dissent. *Communication Studies, 68*(3), 353–367. doi:10.1080.10510974.1334147

Hagiwara, Y., Healy, J., Less, S., Ross, J., Fischer, D., & Sanches-Reily, S. (2018). Development and validation of a Family Meeting Assessment Tool (FMAT). *Journal of Pain and Symptom Management, 55*(1), 89–93. doi:10.1016/j.jpainsymman.2017.07.048

Harrison, C., & Killion, J. (2007). Ten roles for teacher leaders. *Educational Leadership, 65*(1), 74–77.

Hudson, P., Quinn, K., O'Hanlon, B., & Aranda, S. (2008). Family meetings in palliative care: Multidisciplinary clinical practice guidelines. *BMC Palliative Care, 7,* 1–12. doi:10.1186/1472-684X-7-12

Imes, R. S., & Hester, J. (2014). *Loving group work: Is this is Holy Grail of group communication? Investigating a transdisciplinary palliative care team.* Paper presented at the National Communication Association Annual Convention, Chicago, IL.

Imes, R. S., & Hester, J. (2015). *Unintended intentional community at work: Applying a new lens to guide the formation and maintenance of transdisciplinary teams.* Paper presented at the National Communication Association Annual Convention, Las Vegas, NV.

Janis, I. (1982). *Groupthink.* Boston: Houghton Mifflin.

Jehn, K. A. (1995). A multimethod examination of the benefits and detriments of intragroup conflict. *Administrative Science Quarterly, 40,* 256–282. doi:10.2307/2393638

Joint Commission. (2008). Behaviors that undermine a culture of safety. *Sentinel Event Alert,* (40). Retrieved from https://www.jointcommission.org/resources/patient-safety-topics/sentinel-event/sentinel-event-alert-newsletters/sentinel-event-alert-issue-40-behaviors-that-undermine-a-culture-of-safety/

Joint Commission Resources. (2016, December). *Clarification: Use of secure text messaging for patient care orders is not acceptable. Perspectives.* Retrieved from www.jointcommission.org/assets/1/6/Clarification_Use_of_Secure_Text_Messaging.pdf

Kaba, A., & Beran, T. N. (2016). Impact of peer pressure on accuracy of reporting vital signs: Evidence of errors among medical and nursing students in simulations. *Journal of Interprofessional Care, 30*(1), 116–122. doi:10.3109/13561820.2015.1075967

Kaba, A., Wishart, I., Fraser, K., Coderre, S., & McLaughlin, K. (2016). Are we at risk of groupthink in our approach to teamwork interventions in health care? *Medical Education, 50,* 400–408. doi:10.1111/medu.12943

Kauffeld, S., & Lehmann-Willenbrock, N. (2012). Meetings matter: Effects of team meetings on team and organizational success. *Small Group Research, 43*(2), 130–158. doi:10.1177/1046496411429599

Olsen, B., Jason, L. A., Davidson, M., & Ferrari, J. R. (2009). Increases in tolerance within naturalistic, intentional communities: A randomized, longitudinal examination. *American Journal Community Psychology, 44,* 188–195. doi:S10.1007/s10464-009-9275-3

Omilion-Hodges, L. M., & Ackerman, C. D. (2018). From the technical know-how to the free flow of ideas: Exploring the effects of leader, peer, and team communication on employee creativity. *Communication Quarterly, 66*(1), 38–57. doi:10.1080/01463373.2017.1325385

Omilion-Hodges, L. M., & Swords, N. M. (2016). Communication that heals: Mindful communication practices from palliative care leaders. *Health Communication, 31*(3), 328–335. doi:10.1080/10410236.2014.953739

Omilion-Hodges, L. M., & Swords, N. M. (2017). The grim reaper, hounds of hell, and Dr. Death: The role of storytelling for palliative care in competing medical meaning systems. *Health Communication, 32*(10), 1272–1283. doi:10.1080/10410236.2016.1219928

O'Neill, T. A., & Allen, N. J. (2012). Team meeting attitudes: Conceptualization and investigation of a new construct. *Small Group Research, 43*(2), 186–210. doi:10.1177/1046496411426485

Sanders, J. J., Curtis, J. R., & Tulsky, J. A. (2018). Achieving goal-concordant care: A conceptual model and approach to measuring serious illness communication and its impact. *Journal of Palliative Medicine, 21*(S2), 17–24. doi:10.1089/jmp.2017.0459

Shapiro, J., & Nadelman, S. (2014). Support professionalism and trust. In M. Plews-Ogan & G. Beyt (Eds.), *Wisdom leadership in academic health science centers: Leading positive change* (pp. 74–88). London: Radcliffe Publishing.

Sias, P. M., Pederson, H., Gallagher, E. B., & Kopaneva, I. (2012). Workplace friendship in the electronically connected organization. *Human Communication Research, 38*, 253–279. doi:10.1111/j.1468-2958.2012.01428.x

Stevens, D., & Reifsnyder, J. (2018). Improving team effectiveness: Team health and resilience. *Presentation for Center to Advance Palliative Care.* Retrieved from https://www.capc.org/events/recorded-webinars/improving-team-effectiveness-team-health-and-resilience/

Weick, K. (2001). *Making sense of the organization.* Oxford: Blackwell Publishers.

Wyber, R., Khashram, M., Donnell, A., & Meyer-Rochow, G. (2013). The gre8est good: Use of messages between doctors in a tertiary hospital. *Journal of Communication in Healthcare, 6*(1), 29–34. doi:10.1179/1753807612Y.0000000019

CHAPTER 6

OCCUPATIONAL CULTURE: UNDERSTANDING THE ROLE AND STIGMA OF PALLIATIVE CARE

Introduction

High-performing, effective teams do not just happen. Communication and relational complexities underpin the successes or failures of palliative care teams (PCTs). Successful interdisciplinary teams require education and training on teamwork and collaboration, shared goals, specified individual responsibilities, and a clear picture of the interdependence among team roles. While interdisciplinary teams have been praised for their ability to provide holistic patient-centered care and may also help to save money and stave off provider burnout, the various occupational cultures or assumptions of each medical specialty can create unique challenges for the group as a whole. This chapter discusses the communication challenges associated with occupational culture—the ways that various providers have been taught and socialized into practicing medicine and caring for patients. Each medical occupation brings a unique approach to the field and these different approaches have implications for the ways palliative care professionals approach interdisciplinary collaborations. While the demand for palliative care continues to increase, one of the original charges of the specialty—predicting the progression of an illness—has resulted in lingering stigma. Relatedly, tensions between the traditional biomedical model and the more contemporary biopsychosocial model embraced by palliative care professionals result in some organizational challenges. Case in point, some PCT members report that they are referred to as Dr. Death, the grim reaper, or hounds of hell from medical peers in other specialties (Omilion-Hodges & Swords, 2017a). This

---

A podcast to accompany this chapter is available with online access of this title. Please see the instructions on the first page of the book for details on how to access and go to Chapter 6.

illustrates one possible outcome that can emerge when providers from different occupational cultures communicate; however, when done well, interdisciplinary collaboration and teams can enhance patient care.

Negative Palliative Care Experience

Nurse Perspective: Even though I've been here for 32 years, I still have physicians who come up to me and ask "Who have you killed lately?"

Positive Palliative Care Experience

Physician Perspective: I used to think of myself as a cheerleader, but now I just think of myself as the storyteller—the intermediary. I get to know my patients and their families, and many times, they are so appreciative of our services that they ask how to help. I ask for their permission to tell their story, and oftentimes, they will ask "What else?" but once you have a face, a name, and a life to tell, it becomes a lot easier to get approval for the brochures or the physical space or people you need.

Occupational Culture

Every profession brings with it a unique culture. Through an often rigorous educational and training process with numerous testing episodes (e.g., entry to the academic program, theoretical and practical exams, internships, residencies, board exams), individuals are socialized to share beliefs, values, attitudes, and behaviors (Hall, 2005). In addition to shared values, through the educational experiences necessary to become a member, individuals also tend to approach situations similarly and rely on specific language or jargon to do so. Members of occupational communities are defined by four separate, but interconnected, attributes (Van Maanen & Barley, 1984):

- **Boundaries:** Occupations have specific inclusion criteria in terms of training and preparation requirements. Those who are admitted but do not fulfill the requirements or who find themselves at odds with the values and beliefs of an occupation are either asked to leave for not meeting requirements or tend to self-select out of the occupation.
- **Social Identity:** Everyone uses a variety of identity or social markers to define themselves and to describe themselves. For example, one might identify as a palliative care nurse, athlete, avid reader, and parent. Occupations, especially those that require extensive education and training, often compose a large part of our social identity. This part of our identity may become emphasized when we are new in organizations and trying to befriend similar others. Our professions are also emphasized outside of work

when we meet new people or are asked to introduce ourselves. In this sense, our occupational identity is ranked at the same level as our name (i.e., "My name is Jonathan, and I'm a palliative care doctor").

■ **Reference Group:** Students are taught by experts how to interpret, evaluate, think about, and respond to various scenarios. This results in members of the profession sharing values, beliefs, and perceptions that apply to and extend beyond the occupation. The easiest way to see this is in the language or jargon of each profession. The use of jargon has long been an obstacle to interdisciplinary collaboration as different terminology can create confusion and exclude others either intentionally or unintentionally.

■ **Social Relationships:** We often develop and build friendships with colleagues in our profession; this may stem from our shared similarities. Occupational groups can determine who we go to when we have a work-related problem or with whom we sit at lunch. Social relationships may go a step further in occupational communities in terms of how we spend our leisure time. Case in point, Tobias, a palliative care physician from St. Martha's Hospital (pseudonym), suggested that spending time with colleagues and socializing out of work helps providers to cope with the challenges of the job. Relatedly, members of the St. Martha's PCT also text during non-work hours about inside jokes and to coordinate social plans. The social relationships that have emerged among St. Martha's PCT illustrate how members can and often do bond over shared social identity.

Thus, occupational culture not only provides a guide for how to think about and deliver patient care; it also colors our individual identity, who we are likely to befriend and connect with in the workplace, and even how we spend our time outside of work.

How Does Occupational Culture Impact Interdisciplinary Collaboration?

While individuals from different occupations are needed for interdisciplinary teams, the varied educational paths to becoming a member of a specific profession can make interdisciplinary collaboration challenging. From the language used to discuss patient care to approaches to organizing within teams, physicians, nurses, social workers, chaplains, and pharmacists are all likely to take slightly different paths. For example, as many physicians are used to working in highly competitive environments and using assertive or even aggressive communication to take charge of situations, this may be their default manner of communicating and problem-solving.

While this is how some physicians are socialized to demonstrate their expertise in professional settings, it may create an environment that inadvertently makes it

EXHIBIT 6.1

OCCUPATIONAL BOUNDARIES AND PALLIATIVE CARE TEAM DECISION-MAKING

Morning table rounds conversation to coordinate patient care:

APRN: Now, Perry Williams. So right now pulmonary and surg onc are thumb wrestling over the trach. Pulmonary says "He probably needs a trach and we should do it earlier rather than wait the whole weaning." Surg onc says "We do not recommend a trach at this time as we believe he hasn't been fully weaned long enough for intermittent periods of time. We would like to see an attempt at extubation. If he fails this, we will do a trach."

Social Worker: Uh-oh, that's kind of tug-of-war.

APRN: Yep. Surg onc is like "We're out." And pulmonary is like "I'm the pulmonologist."

Social Worker: Yeah. So that's how that's gonna go. So, Perry, is status quo. He's comfortable; his symptoms are under control. His son was supposed to come in, wasn't he?

APRN: I thought so, but I haven't seen him.

Chaplain: I saw him for a few minutes—he was doing better. I'll call to check up while we wait to see what happens between surg onc and pulmonary.

more difficult for other group members to feel comfortable sharing suggestions or alternatives. In some cases, such as the scenario in Exhibit 6.1, team members are waiting for referring physicians to decide on a treatment plan rather than working on the problem as a team. Refer to Box 6.1 for additional examples of team-related outcomes related to various occupational socialization experiences.

Socialization into various medical professions may also include instruction under either the biomedical or biopsychosocial model. While the approaches to medicine of these two models are addressed in greater detail later in this chapter, additional elements that help to support the scaffolding of medical systems—such as hierarchies and status differences—can also create barriers to successful interdisciplinary collaboration.

Historically, physicians have been positioned as the foremost experts in the delivery of patient care. This positioning leads to an implicit (and in some cases, explicit) rank order system where clinicians and caregivers from other occupations (e.g., nursing, social work, and chaplaincy) may feel that their opinions and contributions matter less. Research also indicates that some physicians, particularly

BOX 6.1

SOCIALIZATION INTO VARIOUS OCCUPATIONAL COMMUNITIES

Occupational socialization can lead to different expectations and behaviors based on the profession. These different socialization experiences can create unique challenges for newly formed interdisciplinary teams or for members who are new to interdisciplinary collaboration.

■ Because they are socialized into a culture that stresses confidentiality, *social workers* and *chaplains* in particular may initially feel discomfort in sharing patient information during PCT meetings.

■ *Physicians* often come to the profession through very competitive environments where they often study, learn, and test independently. This pattern of behavior can make it difficult for them to immediately embrace an interdisciplinary approach.

■ *Nurses* are often taught to work within teams as students and as they transition into their careers. This socialization may lead them to be frustrated with team members who have less experience working within teams.

specialists, may be perceived as and taught to see themselves as the expert in rare diseases or surgical interventions and not necessarily in the day-to-day provision of patient health and wellness, such as mental health, common colds, or chronic illnesses (Rose, 2011). While this view is becoming outmoded and is certainly not true of all physicians, empirical research has demonstrated that the rank order system leads to medical errors, even at the epidemic level (Makary & Daniel, 2016). Sutcliffe, Lewton, and Rosenthal (2004) discuss the latent flaws in the medical system that can lead to mishaps and even oversights in patient care. These obstacles include the following:

■ Complex and fragmented healthcare systems
■ Faulty or nonexistent communication
■ Hierarchies and power differences
■ Fear of upward influence
■ Role conflict and ambiguity
■ Interpersonal power struggles
■ Team conflict

As illustrated in Box 6.2, communication challenges are part and parcel with interdisciplinary work.

BOX 6.2

AN RN REFLECTS: I WORK WITH YOU, NOT FOR YOU

The physician I work with is very old school. I've never been invited to call him by his first name and he often refers to me as "my nurse" when talking to others—like I'm his assistant or something. We have a great working relationship, and I know he values my work. I just don't think it has occurred to him that his words make it sound like I work for him rather than with him.

Interdisciplinary Communication

The ability to work effectively in interdisciplinary teams is identified as a core educational competency for all healthcare professionals (Interprofessional Education Collaborative Expert Panel, 2011). Yet a number of systemic challenges make it difficult, if not impossible, for those in the medical field to leave educational systems with a solid foundation and experience in how to develop and facilitate high-performing interdisciplinary and transdisciplinary care teams.

Some of these challenges include the following:

- Lack of time
- Lack of faculty expertise to provide authentic interdisciplinary collaboration experiences
- Cost
- Occupational or governing body accreditation or graduation requirements
- Absence of universal interdisciplinary requirements

At the same time, due to the demand for collaborative care teams, others have gone so far to say that it is no longer appropriate for providers to be trained solely within their respective disciplines (O'Keefe & Ward, 2018). They believe the only way to form high-performing teams is to start from the beginning of the provider educational experience. While the field waits to evolve, teams can learn to be aware of the occupational culture barriers to effective team communication and commit to overcome those deficits (Box 6.3). One way that PCTs and providers may overcome common occupational culture barriers is through storytelling.

BOX 6.3

CHALLENGES ASSOCIATED WITH INTERDISCIPLINARY COMMUNICATION

- When communication skills are addressed in occupational training, the focus is on perspectives and best practices from a specific discipline.

- While students may spend time learning how to communicate with patients and colleagues as a nurse/physician/social worker/chaplain/pharmacist, this does not mean that they are prepared to do so effectively with other occupations.

- New providers not only have to socialize to the profession, but they also have to overcome biases, learn on the job how to integrate various approaches to problem-solving and patient care, and interpret unfamiliar language.

SOURCE: Hall, P. (2005). Interprofessional teamwork: Professional cultures as barriers. *Journal of Interprofessional Care, 19*(Suppl. 1), 188–196. doi:10.1080/13561820500081745

Storytelling

Storytelling is another illustration of the foundational role of communication in meaning making. Storytelling can be a powerful means of establishing palliative care practitioners' agency and in legitimizing the specialty. Omilion-Hodges and Swords (2017a) found that palliative care professionals reported that storytelling helped them to: manage the demands of practicing medicine, navigate team stressors, and advocate for the specialty.

Humans are storytelling creatures; we teach young children how to manage their emotions, how to make good choices, and how to discern good from evil in classic tales that are centuries old. When we meet someone new, many times they will ask in so many words, "What's your story?" The same goes if we are inquiring about someone new from a shared acquaintance: "What's his or her story?" Families, romantic partners, and friends often revisit shared experiences or stories as a means of reaffirming the relationship, as was exemplified by members of St. Martha's PCT telling their origin story in Chapter 3, Formation and Maintenance of

High-Performing Palliative Care Teams. Because we are already predisposed to storytelling, the same principles can help providers in the workplace.

Why Storytelling?

- Stories can serve as sensemaking devices—that is, they can help us to communicate our expertise and specific role responsibilities to others in interdisciplinary and transdisciplinary teams. Weick's (1995, 2005) work in organizational psychology shows us that stories play an important role in *retroactive sensemaking*. In other words, we use stories to help understand our actions, the actions of others, and outcomes. Weick reminds us that organizations are made of massive amounts of data, including everything from budget spreadsheets to the facial expression on a patient who is coming to understand that curing is not going to be a part of his or her journey at this time. Weick also suggested that individuals, dyads, and groups in the organization can reasonably come to different plausible conclusions based on the same data. Storytelling helps teams understand their actions and decision-making in retrospect, and that understanding is used as a part of future actions and decisions.

- Narratives can be rational and/or they can appeal to others' emotions. The best stories will integrate rationality and logic along with a more personal or anecdotal element. For example, when asked why they chose to specialize or work in palliative care, a PCT member may discuss the changing demographics nationwide, the need for holistic care that embraces death as a natural aspect of life, and perhaps a short snippet of a rewarding good death of which they were a part. Members may also choose to share more specific and individual reasons that led them to the specialty.

- Stories help others to feel empathy and encourage perspective taking. Aligning with the foundational role of communication described earlier, palliative care professionals have found that sharing instances of good deaths (with the patient's permission) allowed them to demonstrate the power and scope of their specialty.

- Storytelling results in the creation and stabilization of identities. The more the positive stories that are told about the function and influence of palliative care in patients' lives, the more quickly misconceptions about the specialty are clarified. That is, when family members tell their friends and neighbors of the ways that palliative care is helping their loved ones with serious illnesses or is helping to orchestrate the end-of-life process with dignity, individuals begin to separate it from hospice and see its unique value.

How Do I Tell My Story?

The following section offers suggestions for students and new and seasoned palliative care professionals. The questions provided in Box 6.4 may be a good starting point for considering aspects to integrate into your story.

BOX 6.4

LEARNING ON THE JOB: QUESTIONS AND CONCERNS OFTEN NOT ADDRESSED IN TRAINING PROGRAMS

Some questions that are often not answered or addressed in educational and training programs include the following:

- What shared knowledge, skills, and abilities do my team members and I need to facilitate patient-centered care?

- How do my individual task responsibilities shift, expand, or shrink based on the makeup of the interdisciplinary care team?

- How do my goals as a _____ (nurse/physician/social worker/chaplain/pharmacist) align with my team's purpose and goals?

- How might my goals as a _____ (nurse/physician/social worker/chaplain/pharmacist) diverge from my team's purpose and goals?

- How do I demonstrate my expertise and experience through my communication with my peers?

- How does the way I demonstrate my expertise and experience shift as I communicate with patients and their families?

- How do I demonstrate respect for my colleague(s) when I disagree with them?

- How do I communicate my expectations for how I expect to be treated within the interdisciplinary care team?

- **Students:** Those new to palliative care should focus on the strengths of their particular profession. That is, what makes a nurse, physician, or social worker unique? What skills do they have that other providers may not have? What do chaplains or pharmacists bring to patient care that would otherwise be missing? An initial focus on occupational identity can be a helpful way for students to begin to visualize the specific role they are training for and the concrete ways in which they will be able to ease patient suffering through the care they provide.

- **New Palliative Care Professionals:** New professionals are likely best served by having a prepared elevator pitch about their training and, more importantly, their unique contributions to patient care and interdisciplinary teams. They can assimilate more quickly into teams and new organizations by speaking in assertive, declarative sentences. This means when another member turns and says "What do you bring to the table?" or "What is your story?" instead of being caught off guard or stumbling to articulate a thoughtful response, the new PCT member demonstrates confidence in their reply. This reply should not sound scripted; rather, because of the amount of thought that has gone into who they are as a provider, what they do, and how they approach their work, they are positioned to offer an intentional, but conversational, response. This approach has also been recommended as a way to minimize status differences and guard against medical mishaps (Omilion-Hodges, 2019).

■ **Seasoned Palliative Care Professionals:** While important for students and new PCT members, it may be more natural for seasoned professionals to use powerful communication. Powerful communication does not mean speaking over others or aggressively controlling the conversation; it means that it is important to convince others to listen in situations where one has knowledge, experience, and expertise. This means using declarative sentences and avoiding hedges and justifications. For example, an experienced provider should feel comfortable speaking up in a situation where they believe someone else has made an error, overlooked an aspect of a patient's case, or if the provider would like to suggest an alternative. Thus, a palliative care nurse could demonstrate expertise through powerful communication by saying "The dose prescribed is incorrect given the patient's weight," rather than using powerless language such as "I might be wrong, but this dose doesn't seem correct, does it?" Returning to the foundational role of communication, seasoned providers should practice employing assertive, yet inclusive, language and embracing the responsibility of their experience and position and what that means for their unique contribution to a PCT.

One individual story PCT members consider is their professional arc story; in other words, it is the short story of their careers so far. For some, this story includes the various positions they have held and the organizations for which they have worked. For others, it includes the professions they worked in before finding their way to palliative care (Box 6.5).

Prevailing cultural narratives impact the reception of stories told. For example, the "American Dream" is often narrowly defined as achieving higher and higher levels of administrative responsibility. For those who embrace this definition of success, the story of interdisciplinary teams may ring hollow if they do not have good experiences working in collaborative environments. When informal and formal leadership is valued and all team members work well together, team member satisfaction increases (Lemieux-Charles & McGuire, 2006), and that can be the desired outcome for, and story told about, meaningful work. However, if advancing levels of administrative responsibility are of interest to a team leader because of the perception that success is measured by quickly climbing the hierarchy,

BOX 6.5

A RESIDENT REFLECTS: CHOOSING THE RIGHT SPECIALTY

My internal medicine program was very ICU heavy. By the time I was done, I was feeling like I was doing more harm than good probably. I felt kind of depressed as an intern, which a lot of interns do. You know, you are like … you have the blues, you're just tired, and you feel down; you're the bottom of the totem pole. I started to realize this when there was one patient—she was screaming, and people were holding her down. She had dementia, and I got the procedure done—I put the central line in. I walked out, and I felt like I was going to throw up. And the intensivists and the nurses clapped when I came out of the room because I got the procedure done. And I remember I went home and I called my mom and I said, "This isn't for me." In residency, I started working with the palliative care team more, and I felt like "That's where I want to be." And so I still want to do medicine—I just feel like this is good medicine, not just cookbook medicine.

members may jump to roles that they are not yet ready to do because they feel like it fits their ability to fulfill the story of success in their chosen profession.

Case in point, in the June 14, 2019, GeriPal podcast, Dr. Diane Meier, director of the Center to Advance Palliative Care, cautions newly minted physicians who complete a palliative care fellowship to avoid the seduction of becoming team lead immediately following the completion of their fellowship. She says "Every time I talk to someone who does this, they are in tears." The offer of team lead so early in the professional arc can be flattering—such an achievement adds to the U.S. mythology of the increased value of early success in achieving a position up the hierarchy. However, if the next part of the story is how the frustration of the team lead and the team as a whole could have been lessened by a more experienced leader, neither the new physician nor the team gained much in this story. In fact, if this increased frustration and feelings of helplessness lead to a faster burnout rate, then it becomes a story where everyone loses: the leader, the team, and the patients and their families.

Storytelling can also have a powerful effect on resource allocation in a health system. While quantitative data enumerating clinical, operational, and financial outcomes are crucial for measuring a palliative care program's value, telling patient stories can demonstrate the human side of care. Alongside the numbers, PCT members might consider embedding the "story" of their care to contextualize why those numbers matter. Eliciting a story directly from a patient or family who expresses gratitude for the care received is another way to show the value of your PCT (Box 6.6).

BOX 6.6

A FAMILY MEMBER REFLECTS: THE NECESSITY OF PALLIATIVE CARE

We first met the palliative care team about a year ago when Mom was first hospitalized. At the time, we weren't sure we needed them, but they were invaluable in helping manage Mom's pain when cancer started to take its toll. They also helped her figure out what was most important to her—things like going to her granddaughter's baptism and doing crafts in her own apartment. Mom was a pleaser, and it was really hard for her to tell the oncologist that she didn't want any more chemo because it was making her too sick to do those things. The nurses and social workers and chaplains were like family through the hardest time of our lives. I simply cannot imagine how we would have gotten through this without them. Before Mom died, she asked one of the palliative care NPs what we could do to make sure every cancer patient can get palliative care. The nurse told us it would help to let the oncologist know how important it was and to consider telling our story to hospital administration. My mom made us promise to write the best letter ever, or she'd come back and haunt us.

As shown in earlier chapters, stories about team and individual palliative provider identity are often told in the context of how the PCT is different from other departments in the hospital. The next section considers some common challenges associated with occupational cultures and collaborative care teams.

Tensions Between Palliative Care Providers and Other Medical Providers

Although demand for the specialty continues to increase annually (Center to Advance Palliative Care [CAPC], 2018), palliative care providers often report resistance and peer tension from other medical professionals (Omilion-Hodges & Swords, 2017a). Communication researchers Omilion-Hodges and Swords traced these organizational stressors back to the use of different interpretive models. An interpretive model is a general way of viewing and approaching patient care and how the work of medicine is organized and completed. In other words, it can give providers a general sense of meaning for how to practice their profession. Because interpretive models provide a set of guiding beliefs and guidelines for practice, interpretive models are often intertwined with occupational culture training and education. In many ways, these models help to answer the question of how care providers (physicians, nurses, social workers, etc.) provide care in their occupation.

There are two predominate models in medicine: the traditional biomedical model of medicine that privileges curative treatment and the biopsychosocial model of medicine that emphasizes holistic care (Figure 6.1). Though these models should work in concert and borrow standardized processes from one another when helpful, more commonly they spark deep divides between specialties and wedge tension between providers (Omilion-Hodges & Swords, 2017a,b). This may stem from the clear distinctions and the fact that various occupations are often instructed in different models.

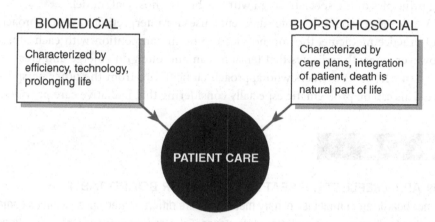

BIOMEDICAL

Characterized by efficiency, technology, prolonging life

BIOPSYCHOSOCIAL

Characterized by care plans, integration of patient, death is natural part of life

PATIENT CARE

FIGURE 6.1 Biomedical versus biopsychosocial model.

Biomedical Model of Medicine

- Traditional approach, in Western medicine, to organizing and delivering care
- Stresses the guiding and expert voice of the physician, a treatment plan, efficiency, and technological innovations and interventions
- Clear focus on the extension of life
- Death or patients who are no longer responsive to treatment may be interpreted as a failure of a provider

Recent research (Omilion-Hodges & Swords, 2017a) found that providers in cardiology, neurology, and oncology may still be trained and operate under this model—especially considering that these specialties often deal in rare interventions and may secure a competitive advantage over other healthcare centers based on their cutting-edge technology.

Biopsychosocial Model of Medicine

- Contemporary approach to viewing the role of medicine in patient care
- Integrates patients' wishes, their lifestyle, and their family into a holistic care plan
- Emphasizes family, individualized communication, and active listening
- Embraces death as a natural aspect of life

As palliative care is founded on the notion that it takes an interdisciplinary team to help those with serious illnesses or who are near the end of life, the guiding principles of the specialty align with the biopsychosocial model.

While these two models offer different lenses for interpreting how to approach and practice medicine, they do not need to be in competition with each other. However, research indicates that tensions can and often do emerge and create a division between providers who approach clinical care from the other perspective. This can be problematic especially considering that palliative care providers

BOX 6.7

AN APRN REFLECTS: A SEAT AT THE TUMOR BOARD TABLE

Tumor boards are a multidisciplinary meeting where different medical specialties come together to discuss cases and share knowledge. For a cancer program, these meetings are an important part of care because they bring together all of the experts to come up with the best treatment plan. Palliative care can offer a valuable perspective but may not be explicitly invited to participate. If you find yourself sitting on the edge of the discussion, here are some strategies to integrate palliative care into a multidisciplinary meeting like tumor boards:

- Show up—consistently.
- Sit at the table or the front of the room.
- Review cases prior to the meeting in order to be prepared to speak to potential palliative care issues and needs.
- Speak up, especially when palliative care is already involved in the case. This will demonstrate the value that palliative care has already added to the patient's care.
- Be sure to align with other specialists: "How can I help support this treatment plan?"
- Offer to present cases.

and teams tend to operate from a biopsychosocial stance. The distinction between the two may become clearer when an oncology patient, for example, is no longer responding to curative treatment and the attending oncologist communicates with (or neglects to communicate with) the PCT to coordinate care. Box 6.7 is an example of how PCTs may preemptively become involved in easing the distinction between the models to enhance patient care while elevating the profile of the team.

Contemporary Tensions Palliative Care Providers Commonly Navigate

Stemming from the differences in the biomedical and the biopsychosocial approaches to medicine, providers from nationally award-winning palliative care units (American Hospital Association, n.d.) report navigating two primary tensions: living–dying and practicing–advocating. Tensions such as these never disappear; rather, individuals find ways of addressing the challenges as relationships grow and evolve.

In addition to the two tensions that palliative care providers navigate frequently, other pressures that medical providers often face include cure-cure and leading-following (Considine & Miller, 2010).

Tension 1: Living–Dying

This tension emerges from the perceived conflict between the focus of palliative care and that of the rest of the medical community. On one side, there resides the objective of virtually all medical specialties—that healthcare professionals work to prolong life. Though the goal of palliative care is not the opposing side—dying—others in both the medical and lay community often interpret it as such. This may be because the original purpose of palliative care was designed to predict how a patient's illness would progress based on the original diagnosis (Rokach, 2005). This tension is also thought to arise from the divergence from the traditional biomedical model. Because the biomedical lens has been the default approach for decades and this approach has always stressed prolonging life, it may be particularly challenging for the larger medical community to shift to embracing death as a natural aspect of life. Relatedly, the biomedical approach focuses on treatment plans in contrast to the biopsychosocial focus on care plans. As Margaret, a palliative care physician, put it, "Most physicians treat diseases, not people," also suggesting that "it's impossible to communicate comprehensively about end-of-life care

BOX 6.8

PALLIATIVE CARE PROVIDERS REFLECT ON COMMON ORGANIZATIONAL TENSIONS

Exemplifying the Living–Dying Tension

■ **Christopher, a palliative care physician:**

Everyone passes away. It's an honor to spend that time with patients and their families and to help them through the process. What I don't understand is that when they [other physicians] or a loved one approach[es] end of life, this is exactly what [they] will seek (p. 1278).

Exemplifying the Practicing–Advocating Tension

■ **Jameson, a pediatric palliative care physician:**

I wish that others understood what I really do. In addition to monitoring a patient and tending to their physical needs and helping to manage their pain, I get to know them. I ask them questions. I don't set a broken arm and then send the patient away—I become part of the family and treat them all (p. 1278).

SOURCE: Quotes drawn from Omilion-Hodges, L. M., & Swords, N. M. (2017a). The grim reaper, hounds of hell, and Dr. Death: The role of storytelling for palliative care leaders in competing medical meaning systems. *Health Communication, 32*(10), 1272–1283. doi:10.1080/10410236.2016 .1219928

or options if you don't know what to do in the absence of a treatment plan" (Omilion-Hodges & Swords, 2017a, p. 1276); for more provider reflections, refer to Box 6.8.

Considering this, PCTs must navigate this occupational tension within the workplace and community, as they strive to care for patients (Box 6.9). More specifically, because this tension involves a lack of clarity or care surrounding learning the nuances of palliative care, it has clear consequences for peer relationships and may color the way the healthcare facility and surrounding community view the local PCT. Research has found that the lack of understanding can stem from knowledge, communication, and value gaps (Omilion-Hodges & Swords, 2017a). While it seems unlikely, these gaps can even be experienced by those who understand palliative care when it is their own loved ones who are seriously ill (Box 6.10).

BOX 6.9

A PHYSICIAN REFLECTS: TEACHING COLLEAGUES ABOUT PALLIATIVE CARE

I entered an order for fluids for a patient with a UTI. My order was ignored. I went to the bedside nurse and asked why he didn't hang the IV for the patient, and he said "She is in palliative. Why would she need IV fluids?" I was stunned. The patient was in pain and dehydrated. We could help her with both of those, and she wanted the help. When I explained to this to the nurse, he said "We are helping. She's in palliative, so that means she doesn't want any more treatment for anything."

BOX 6.10

A CHAPLAIN REFLECTS: CARING FOR THE FAMILY MEMBERS OF HEALTHCARE PROVIDERS

Recently, the palliative care team was consulted on the critically ill wife of one of our hospital's pulmonologists. The nurses in the ICU were worried that he was getting too involved in daily medical decisions—micromanaging the residents and even the attendings at times. While this pulmonologist consults palliative care often for his patients, he waved us off for his wife, saying "You guys are great, but she's going to be fine." Even though he wouldn't let us get involved in her case, I made sure to let him know that I was praying for his wife's healing whenever I saw him in the hall. Eventually, he broke down and told me that he felt like he was failing as a physician and as a husband because he couldn't make her better. I suggested that he might let some of his most trusted colleagues wear the doctor hat for a while so he could focus on being a husband, pointing out that the whole medical team was replaceable to his wife, but he was not. He let us in at that point, and we worked hard to explicitly honor his medical knowledge while carving out emotional space for him to tend to his wife as a loved one.

Tension 2: Practicing–Advocating

Palliative care practitioners may find themselves in the position of having to explain the nuances of their specialty, how it differs from hospice, and why and how an interdisciplinary care team can help to improve quality of life during treatment or to facilitate a good death. Thus, unlike other specialties such as obstetrics and cardiology whose scope and role tend to be clear to patients and are long established in the medical field, palliative care providers may have to do double duty in terms of delivering care and advocating for the profession. Madeline, a palliative care physician, explained that "cardiologists don't actively persuade others of the value of their services or have to explain what cardiology means or what cardiologists do" (pp. 1278–1279).

Palliative care providers have found that the use of intentional communication in the form of storytelling helps them to successfully navigate the practicing–advocating tension (see the "Storytelling" section). Practicing palliative care professionals will likely recognize that they already use this communication skill in terms of discussing patient stories (with the patients' permission, of course). Providers may also enact elements of storytelling with patients in reviewing their medical histories and emphasizing shared similarities as a means of developing rapport (Omilion-Hodges & Swords, 2016).

Having discussed the challenging tensions of the two predominate approaches to medical care, the next section considers how this intersection can impact the daily work lives of palliative care professionals.

Putting It All Together: How Varied Approaches to Medicine and Occupational Culture Impact Palliative Care Providers and Teams

Various ways of thinking about and practicing clinical care can impact peer relationships, the relationship a PCT shares with the healthcare facility, and also the relationship a PCT shares with the community as a whole. This section emphasizes some of the more challenging encounters that palliative care providers have experienced, particularly because the focus of the occupation is often misunderstood. Additionally, as palliative care professionals view death as a natural part of life, tensions can arise when other medical professionals have been socialized to create treatment plans and utilize the newest technological interventions to sustain a patient's life as long as possible.

Challenges in Interdisciplinary Peer Relationships

Interdisciplinary relationships can be difficult to navigate even when providers are operating from the same medical model. Misunderstandings can arise from providers in different occupations using profession-specific language or jargon,

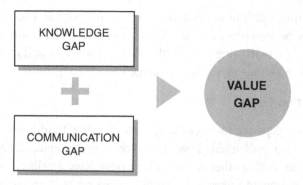

FIGURE 6.2 Visual representation of knowledge, communication, and value gaps.

taking different approaches to providing patient care and in negotiating hierarchy and/or power differences. Considering this, it becomes even more apparent why forging high-functioning, two-way communicative relationships across disciplines can be daunting.

Knowledge, communication, and *value gaps* may help to explain some of the stress palliative care providers have incurred in their interactions with other medical peers (Figure 6.2). For example, a number of palliative care providers acknowledge semi-routine name calling from peers in other medical specialties. Even practitioners from units who have been awarded the American Hospital Association Circle of Life Award reveal that they and their teams are commonly called the death squad, angels of death, grim reapers, and the hounds of hell (Omilion-Hodges & Swords, 2017a, p. 1276). These unfortunate and unprofessional instances of name calling may stem from a knowledge gap.

Knowledge Gaps

Knowledge gaps are surface-level misunderstandings that may include medical colleagues not understanding the scope and focus of palliative care and/or the general discomfort that attending physicians may feel when they refer a patient to palliative care. Though it can be delivered in concert with curative treatment, many medical providers outside of the discipline may be accustomed to only thinking about palliative care when a patient stops responding to treatment options. Steven, a palliative care physician, has found that he and/or members of his team are often in the unfortunate position of having to break the news to patients and their families that they were not released to his palliative care facility "to build strength." In other words, a number of Steven's patients are not told by their attending physicians that they are no longer candidates for curative measures. Since knowledge gaps emerge from a lack of understanding of the purpose and scope of palliative care, they may be lessened through learning opportunities. Continuing medical education courses, marketing and/or educational materials, and interdisciplinary peer retreats or meetings may help to assuage knowledge gaps.

Communication Gaps

Communication gaps are more challenging to alleviate than knowledge gaps, as they presume that individuals have a surface-level understanding of palliative care. This may mean that other providers have completed a palliative care, hospice, or geriatrics rotation and have some exposure to a realistic understanding of the specialty. Ahmed, a palliative care nurse, saw communication gaps as "an outsider's stereotypes of the profession" (Omilion-Hodges & Swords, 2017a, p. 1277). Yet despite the experience or general understanding of the discipline, individuals may remain unaware of the nuances of the profession and, worst yet, know and communicate just enough about palliative care to be dangerous. What is meant by this is that while medical professionals may be able to nuance palliative care from hospice care, they may not be able to give accurate or realistic information to colleagues, patients, or a general audience about the breadth of services palliative care providers offer, typical occupational makeup of PCTs, or how the discipline is billed and operates with private pay insurances or Medicare.

Value Gaps

Value gaps are the most burdensome assumptions or occupational misunderstandings to shake. Research with a nationwide sample of palliative care providers revealed that since the specialty embraces death as a natural aspect of life, other medical providers may feel that their specialty requires more training, skill, or fortitude as a means of saving or extending life. Value gaps also include the challenges associated with knowledge and communication gaps. The compounding of misconceptions and stereotypes are what make value gaps so harmful. That is, regardless of the amount of information someone has about the specialty, it is unlikely that they will come to view palliative care as an essential aspect of medical care. Common questions that characterize value gaps in palliative care include the following (Omilion-Hodges & Swords, 2017a, p. 1277):

■ Why do I need a doctor to help me die?
■ Why are there death doctors?
■ Everyone dies. So what do you do?

See Box 6.11 for examples of knowledge, communication, and value gaps.

BOX 6.11

EXAMPLES OF KNOWLEDGE, COMMUNICATION, AND VALUE GAPS

Knowledge gap: "I actually had one oncologist tell me that since I'm Dr. Death he'll leave that part [communicating about life expectancy] to me," Steven, palliative care physician (p. 1276).

Communication gap: Decorating a palliative care unit as a graveyard during Halloween, complete with a scythe and black cloak, reflects "the deep-rooted lack of understanding of the specialty and a steadfast fear of death among other physicians," Jim, a palliative care physician (p. 1276).

Value gap: Giving a palliative care provider a list of counselor referrals and money intended to be used to secure mental health referrals, complete with a note that says "Don't go postal, Reaper. We're bailing you out," Thomas, a palliative care physician (p. 1277).

SOURCE: Quotes drawn from Omilion-Hodges, L. M., & Swords, N. M. (2017a). The grim reaper, hounds of hell, and Dr. Death: The role of storytelling for palliative care leaders in competing medical meaning systems. *Health Communication, 32*(10), 1272–1283. doi:10.1080/10410236.2016 .1219928

Contradictory Views of Death

If we return to the arduous process of socializing into an occupation, we can see how different providers begin to work within a specific medical model. Considering the time it takes to complete coursework and practical experience requirements to become a certified nurse, physician, social worker, and so forth, it becomes easier to see that by the time providers are integrated into healthcare facilities and care teams, they have long been taught to interpret medicine and deliver care in very specific ways. Thus, if providers have always been instructed explicitly or implicitly that death is a type of failure—either because of provider oversight, medicine, and treatment shortcomings or because the patient did not follow the prescribed treatment plan—then it becomes very challenging to adopt a view of death as a natural aspect of life. Many medical professionals may view death as having not met their goal or that of their patients in terms of allowing them to extend life. Yet, with the rise in patient-centered care and acceptance of the biopsychosocial model, more providers—especially those in palliative care—may engage in conversations with patients and their loved ones about shifting focus from cure to care.

In an editorial (Miller, 2012), a palliative care nurse shared the story of a young mother who decided to stop life-prolonging oncology treatments because the tumor was not significantly shrinking and because the effects of the treatments left her sick, lethargic, and unable to engage with her family in the way she wanted to. Though it was a wrenching decision and challenging for her family to accept initially, embracing non-life-prolonging measures allowed the young woman to enjoy the remainder of her life on her terms. This was seen as a good death by the PCT, the patient, and her family—though this same decision is likely to be viewed less positively by providers who have been trained and worked to extend life (Omilion-Hodges & Swords, 2017b).

Palliative care providers have been quick to recognize that the occasional ill treatment from medical peers is not necessarily rooted in malice, but in fear and grief. Physicians in other specialties may use sarcastic and disparaging humor as a way to deal with the uncomfortable feelings they are experiencing when they realize that one of their patients is approaching end of life.

> It [disrespectful treatment] come[s] to a head when they've just released someone to my care—especially if it's a patient they've been with a while. I know that they're [the physicians] hurting, but telling me 'it's my time to pretend you're useful' is not the optimal way to ask me to care for a patient.—Madeline, a palliative care physician. (Omilion-Hodges & Swords, 2017a, p. 1278)

Organizational and Community Challenges That Palliative Care Teams Face

Just as challenges may arise in interdisciplinary peer interactions, PCTs may find themselves navigating challenges at the organizational and community levels. Since the biomedical model has been the predominate approach for thinking about, organizing, and delivering medicine, it will take time for providers, educational and medical organizations, and community members to gain comfort with another approach (the biopsychosocial model).

Tensions may manifest at the organizational level concerning allotment of resources (refer to Boxes 6.12 and 6.13 for suggestions for what PCTs and providers should negotiate). Because the nonpalliative care approach has historically prized divisions that integrated the latest high-tech innovations and revenue generation, these have often received more resources in the form of funding to secure new technology, new hires trained in the latest innovations, and promotion in the form of ideal office locations (to facilitate patient ease and comfort) and additional attention in terms of marketing collateral (i.e., webpage space, location, brochures, television, and radio ads).

BOX 6.12

WHAT SHOULD PALLIATIVE CARE TEAMS NEGOTIATE FOR?

Ideal physical location: Patients and families in need of palliative care are already negotiating the confusion and complexity associated with serious illness or end of life. A centralized location for designated palliative care units not only is beneficial for patients but also illustrates the organization's support for the specialty. Additionally, PCTs should be afforded adequate office space that allows team members to convene and collaborate together throughout the day when they are not directly caring for patients.

Marketing assistance: Palliative care professionals should get to know their organization's marketing and public relations team members. Doing so allows PCT members to connect with the local community to educate them about the breadth of palliative care and to form relationships. PCTs should also request brochures describing their services, dedicated space on the organization's website, and routine features in internal and external newsletters. Because the focus of palliative care naturally aligns with many health organizations' mission statements, the specialty is ripe to be highlighted for their own mission moments by sharing care stories that align with the guiding principles of the organization.

Systematic new hires: New PCTs and even established teams should consider presenting senior leadership with data concerning the continued rapid rise of the specialty. CAPC (www.capc.org) publishes trends annually. Bringing empirical evidence of the sustained nationwide trend can help providers to secure frequent new hires to keep up with patient demand.

Funding for team and provider development: Developing and maintaining a high-performing team is challenging—this challenge is compounded when members come from different occupations as they do in palliative care. For one high-performing PCT, part of the reason they are so successful as a transdisciplinary team is because they took (and still take) time to identify team guidelines and rules for meetings and are committed to intentional interpersonal communication. This means that they spend time together as people (such as shared daily lunch breaks), not just coworkers, and when conflict arises, they address it swiftly and with transparency. Earmarking PCT money for peer retreats, lunches, and team building activities can help to facilitate stronger team relationships, which can aid in patient-centered care. Moreover, money should be requested on an annual basis for travel, registration, and resources related to professional development in the form of conference attendance, workshop participation, or the ability to purchase new books and resource materials for all disciplines.

A seat at the decision-making table: Palliative care teams should know the procedure for securing a line item on a senior leadership or board of directors meeting agenda. Whether it is to share a particularly moving case that demonstrates a mission moment or to present the latest programmatic and nationwide trends, palliative care leaders should be clear on how to secure the attention of these audiences when necessary.

BOX 6.13

A CHANGE IN ORGANIZATIONAL CULTURE: PHYSICAL CHANGE IN LOCATION FOR ONE PALLIATIVE CARE TEAM

Some palliative care programs have found that organizational resource allocation is shifting to create or augment programs, including moving palliative care units to highly coveted, high-traffic areas that are easy to find, such as near hospital cafeterias and gift shops. Considering the confusion and fear patients with serious illness or near end-of-life feel, having the palliative care unit in an easy-to-access area indicates that organizations are embracing the public demand for the occupation.

While tangible gains are being made at the organizational and community levels to elevate the position of palliative care, this can also create turmoil between medical specialties. Kelly, a chief executive officer and former practicing palliative care physician, shared a fitting example:

> This other doctor, a neurologist, could not ... rationalize why the organization would give money to a program that was not revenue generating. The problem with this, is that making money is prized over an ethical obligation. I didn't become a doctor to make an organization rich. I went into palliative care because caring for people is the right thing to do. (Omilion-Hodges & Swords, 2017a, p. 1277)

Kelly's experience illustrates that, because the demand for palliative care was so great, her organization shifted and allocated more resources to her unit. Though this may seem subtle, with time, these shifts reiterate the importance of viewing death as a natural aspect of life—reinforcing the specialty of palliative care and the larger biopsychosocial model.

SOURCE: Omilion-Hodges, L. M., & Swords, N. M. (2017a). The grim reaper, hounds of hell, and Dr. Death: The role of storytelling for palliative care leaders in competing medical meaning systems. *Health Communication, 32*(10), 1272–1283. doi:10.1080/10410236.2016.1219928

The impact on PCTs by an organization's structural culture can be explained by structurational divergence theory (Nicotera & Clinkscales, 2010; Nicotera et al., 2015; see Figure 6.3). Anderson (2015) points out that the "overall ideology of teamwork amongst and between physicians and nurses is disrupted by an organizational focus on separation" (p. 173). This theory describes the tensions that arise when organizational members are expected to follow two sets of incompatible expectations and this can be expanded from physicians and nurses to the entire PCT. On one hand, all organizational members are expected to be good stewards of hospital resources—in other words, do more with less. On the other hand, as the demand for palliative care continues to skyrocket (CAPC, 2018), a PCT's patient volume continues to grow and the expectation for time-intensive patient-centered care remains the same. This creates structurational divergence. As separation of disciplines has long been the norm for hospitals, the desired move to team-based healthcare may not be met with a cultural change that encourages and supports interdisciplinary teams. If structurational divergence is not managed, teams see greater turnover as frustrated members leave for other positions or leave the practice of palliative care for a different profession.

Great Palliative Care Teams Survive Difficult Organizational Environments

The struggles with organizational obstacles and the stigma for PCTs can be significant. However, due to the vital work PCTs do for patients with serious illness and their families, looking for solutions to help PCTs thrive is worth the effort. As demonstrated in previous chapters, teams built with intention and maintained with thoughtfulness and skill have an excellent chance of surviving difficulties in organizational culture. Over time, the existence of PCTs may come to alter the organizational culture in a way that better cares for patients in a holistic manner. Their example of intentional communication with one another, hospital leadership, patients and families, and other departments in the hospital may lead others to want to do the same.

Embracing the foundational role of communication (see Chapter 1, Why We Need to Talk About Teams and Communication in Palliative Care) can help providers to successfully and tactfully navigate common organizational stressors. Though it may seem simple, focusing on intentional language usage, active listening, and employing an other-oriented and meaning-centered approach can make common organizational stressors all but disappear. Utilizing effective communication empowers providers to own and enact their expertise in a way that honors their knowledge and experience, while facilitating high-performing workgroup relationships with others.

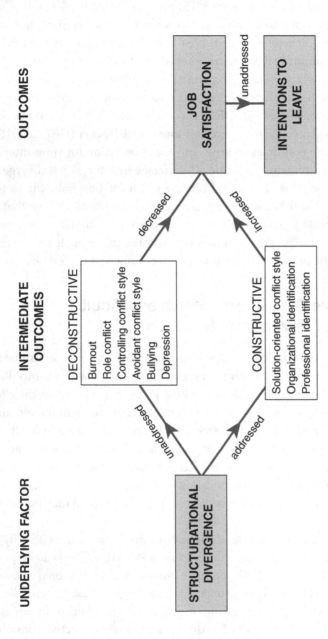

FIGURE 6.3 Structurational divergence outcomes.

SOURCE: Nicotera, A. M., Zhao, X., Mahon, M. M., Peterson, E. B., Kim, W., & Conway-Morana, P. (2015). Structurational divergence theory as explanation for troublesome outcomes in nursing communication. *Health Communication, 30*(4), 371–384. doi:10.1080/10410236.2013.863139

PEARLS FROM THE FIELD: PROVIDER AND TEAM TAKEAWAYS

Building and maintaining high-performing PCTs requires the ongoing hard work of uniting providers from various backgrounds and the lingering tensions between the traditional biomedical model and the more contemporary biopsychosocial model. This means that simple knowledge gaps or more complicated value gaps can interject "noise" into conversations, which may alter or interfere with meaning and interpretation. Three key takeaways are discussed in the following.

Takeaway 1: Occupational culture can help to facilitate socialization into a profession, but it can also inadvertently hinder interdisciplinary communication and collaboration.

Communication with friends, family members, and romantic partners can be challenging—and these are people we generally like! All kidding aside, communication is not always easy and becomes even more complicated in high-stress, high-stakes environments and across occupations.

Though interdisciplinary training is recommended as a best practice for palliative care professionals in training, time limitations, accreditation restrictions, and the inability of faculty to find or create authentic experiences for students mean that many new providers have limited or no firsthand experience in transdisciplinary teams. In some ways, this implies that it should be easy or natural to immediately integrate successfully into a high-performing transdisciplinary team. This puts additional stress on new providers, as they transition into patient care. However, by focusing on the foundational role of communication and practicing the storytelling techniques covered in this chapter, providers will be better positioned to flex communicatively. This means that by enacting the elements of the foundational role of communication and focusing on individual roles, shared team goals, and patient care, new providers will likely experience a smoother integration into the profession, the team, and the workplace.

Takeaway 2: Being a palliative care professional or team member is rewarding, but it is not easy.

The sustained increase in palliative care programs indicates demand and increased legitimacy of the specialty. However, palliative care professionals are still having to correct basic misconceptions about the specialty, even with peers in the medical field. Relatedly, PCT members may be on the receiving end of name calling as an outcome of the two predominate tensions they experience: living–dying and practicing–advocating. These organizational challenges may

(continued next page)

sprout from the differences between the biomedical and biopsychosocial models, the confusion surrounding the breadth and scope of the specialty, and/or the fear and grief other providers experience when a patient they have been caring for is no longer benefiting from life-prolonging treatment.

Despite these challenges, the numbers speak for the specialty. Palliative care is here to stay; it fills a clear gap in medical care and, perhaps more importantly, helps those who are dealing with the confusion and stress of serious illnesses and at end of life.

Takeaway 3: Storytelling is key.

Successful palliative care teams use storytelling to define themselves in ways that demonstrate their worth to the larger organization. The beauty of storytelling is that it is free and it integrates rationality with emotions. PCTs and providers can talk about their high patient census while also highlighting a particular powerful story of a good death. This approach may resonate with hospital and healthcare center administrators, as it quantifies patient demand while exemplifying via a good death story why the demand is as high as it is. Moreover, storytelling can be used to help teach other medical peers about the ins and outs of palliative care. For example, if a PCT realizes a certain oncologist's patients are often unaware that they are no longer candidates for life-sustaining treatment, the team lead may go and share a story of how other attendings tactfully break the news to patients. Finally, storytelling can be a powerful tool for individual providers, as they train, enter the field, and grow in their expertise. Taking time to reflect on one's career arc can help in developing a thoughtful response to the ubiquitous "What do you do?" question. Considering that palliative care is delivered through interdisciplinary teams, providers may find themselves responding to that question frequently in the workplace.

References

American Hospital Association. (n.d.). *Circle of life award: Celebrating innovation in palliative and end-of-life care.* Retrieved from https://www.aha.org/about/awards/circle-life

Anderson, L. (2015). Understanding hospital-based nurses' experiences of structurational divergence. *The Qualitative Report, 20*(3), 172–185.

Center to Advance Palliative Care. (2018). *Palliative care continues its annual growth trend, according to latest center to advance palliative care analysis* [Press release]. Retrieved fromhttps://www.capc.org/about/press-media/press-releases/2018-2-28/palliative-care

-continues-its-annual-growth-trend-according-latest-center-advance-palliative-care
-analysis/

Considine, J., & Miller, K. (2010). The dialectics of care: Communicative choices at the end of life. *Health Communication, 25,* 165–174. doi:10.1080/10410230903544951

Hall, P. (2005). Interprofessional teamwork: Professional cultures as barriers. *Journal of Interprofessional Care, 19*(Suppl. 1), 188–196. doi:10.1080/13561820500081745

Interprofessional Education Collaborative Expert Panel. (2011). *Core competencies for interprofessional collaborative practice: Report of an expert panel.* Washington, DC: Interprofessional Education Collaborative.

Lemieux-Charles, L., & McGuire, W. L. (2006). What do we know about health care team effectiveness: A review of the literature. *Medical Care Research and Review, 63*(3), 263–300. doi:10.1177/1077558706287003

Makary, M. A., & Daniel, M. (2016). Medical error—The third leading cause of death in the US. *BMJ, 353,* i2139.

Meier, D. (2019). *The future of palliative care: A Podcast with Diane Meier.* GeriPal Podcast. Retrieved from https://www.geripal.org/2019/06/the-future-of-palliative-care-podcast_14.html

Miller, E. T. (2012). Care vs cure? *Rehabilitation Nursing, 37,* 161–162. doi:10.1002/rnj.52

Nicotera, A. M., & Clinkscales, M. J. (2010). Nurses at the nexus: A case study in structurational divergence. *Health Communication, 25,* 32–49. doi:10.1080/10410230903473516

Nicotera, A. M., Zhao, X., Mahon, M. M., Peterson, E. B., Kim, W., & Conway-Morana, P. (2015). Structurational divergence theory as explanation for troublesome outcomes in nursing communication. *Health Communication, 30*(4), 371–384. doi:10.1080/10410236.2013.863139

O'Keefe, M., & Ward, H. (2018). Implementing interprofessional learning curriculum: How problems might also be answers. *BMC Medical Education, 18,* 132–240. doi:10.1186/s12909-018-1231-1

Omilion-Hodges, L. M. (2019). A communication-based approach to safeguarding against medical errors. In F. Allhoff & S. L. Borden (Eds.), *Ethics and error in medicine* (pp. 71–86). New York: Routledge.

Omilion-Hodges, L. M., & Swords, N. M. (2016). Communication that heals: Mindful communication practices from palliative care leaders. *Health Communication, 31*(3), 328–335. doi:10.1080/10410236.2014.953739

Omilion-Hodges, L. M., & Swords, N. M. (2017a). The grim reaper, hounds of hell, and Dr. Death: The role of storytelling for palliative care leaders in competing medical meaning systems. *Health Communication, 32*(10), 1272–1283. doi:10.1080/10410236.2016.1219928

Omilion-Hodges, L. M., & Swords, N. M. (2017b). Communication matters: Exploring the intersection of family and provider end of life communication. *Journal of Behavioral Sciences, 7*(1), 15–25. doi:10.3390/bs7010015

Rokach, A. (2005). Caring for those who care for the dying: Coping with the demands on palliative care workers. *Palliative & Supportive Care, 3,* 325–332. doi:10.1017/S1478951505050492

Rose, L. (2011). Interprofessional collaboration in the ICU: How to define? *Nursing In Critical Care, 16,* 5–10. doi:10.1111/j.1478-5153.2010.00398.x

Sutcliffe, K. M., Lewton, E., & Rosenthal, M. M. (2004). Communication failures: An insidious contributor to medical mishaps. *Academic Medicine, 79,* 186–194. doi:10.1097/00001888-200402000-00019

Van Maanen, J., & Barley, S. R. (1984). Occupational communities: Culture and control in organizations. In B. M. Staw & L. L. Cummings (Eds.), *Research in organizational behaviour* (pp. 287–365). Greenwhich, CT: JAI Press.

Weick, K. (1995). *Sensemaking in organizations*. Thousand Oaks, CA: Sage.

Weick, K. (2005). Managing the unexpected: Complexity as distributed sensemaking. In R. R. McDaniel & D. J. Dreibe (Eds.), *Uncertain and surprise in complex systems: Question on working with the unexpected* (pp. 51–78). Berlin: Springer-Verlag.

CHAPTER 7

SELF-CARE AND TEAM CARE IN EMOTIONAL LABOR–INTENSIVE POSITIONS

Introduction

Palliative care is challenging, yet rewarding work. The specialty falls beneath the umbrella of emotional labor–intensive positions. This means that in addition to job-specific responsibilities and duties, palliative care members are often in the position where they must fulfill role requirements while also managing and regulating their own emotions. While employees in most positions have to do this, palliative care is considered emotional labor because it revolves around providing comfort and care to those with serious and terminal illnesses. In this field, healthcare professionals are constantly exposed to others' emotional and physical suffering, which often leads to death and bereavement. Thus, even when team members lose a patient, they are expected to carry out duties throughout their shift. This requires special and intense emotional work to mask one's true emotions with emotions that are expected by peers and patients. This chapter discusses self-care and team care, and debunks misconceptions about working in emotionally intense positions. In the absence of self-care, palliative care professionals become even more susceptible to burnout and compassion fatigue.

Negative Palliative Care Experience

APRN Perspective: I went into this work because of my deep commitment to caring for people who are suffering. Lately, I never leave work on time, and I end up doing half of my charting at home. I feel like there will never be enough hours in the day, and I'm not serving anybody—my patients, my team, or my family. I used to look for chances to really engage with my patients, to find and address the sources of their

---

A podcast to accompany this chapter is available with online access of this title. Please see the instructions on the first page of the book for details on how to access and go to Chapter 7.

suffering. Today, by the time I got to a patient's room, the family had already left. The nurse told me they are really struggling, but what I found myself thinking was "Thank goodness they already left so I can go chart." I don't even recognize myself anymore.

Positive Palliative Care Experiences

Chief Executive Officer Perspective: We signed up for this, and we know what it's [the dying process] like, but it's vital we don't take that for granted when interacting with those we serve.

Physician Perspective: You reach a point where psychologically you have to mark that space off for yourself, where you've got other activities that you do not neglect. Then you're not so immersed in this 24-7 that you lose sight of some of the other things that are happening. But you do have cases that are very touching and trying and that stick with you. You know? The ones that are as vivid now as they were 2 years ago. You have that, and it's just part of the nature of the work, too. I don't know what everybody else does for their own release for that, but I suspect that knowing how it [our team] has played out over time is each one of us probably does have pretty effective ways of coping and dealing with that emotional intensity in an ongoing way.

Emotional Labor–Intensive Positions

Palliative care typifies emotional work. Healthcare professionals use "their selves therapeutically to provide a healing presence to patients in life-threatening crises while simultaneously providing a means for healthcare professionals to cope when facing frequent losses" (Sans et al., 2015, p. 204). In other words, palliative care professionals and teams are instruments of healing but are, at the same time, vulnerable to emotional and pragmatic challenges associated with the profession (Mehta et al., 2016; Sanchez-Reilly et al., 2013).

In emotional labor–intensive positions, employees experience and demonstrate authentic emotional reactions as part of their occupational role (Miller, 2007). Healthcare professionals must then manage and regulate their emotions in normative ways that align with patient and organizational expectations. This means PCT members are expected to demonstrate authentic care and concern when engaging with patients and their families and while carrying out role responsibilities even when experiencing personal grief, such as in the case of losing a special patient. This can be particularly challenging when certain situations or patients look to you "to be a 'person' before a 'medical provider'" (Omilion-Hodges & Swords, 2016, p. 332), yet you are expected to put on a brave and professional front.

BOX 7.1

EXPLORING MEANINGFUL WORK

Many in emotional labor-intensive positions describe their occupations as a calling or as meaningful work. They find a strong sense of purpose and meaning in their role.

In these cases, PCT members may answer the "who am I" question via their occupation. Their professional identity aligns so closely with their personal beliefs and values that they merge into a larger, shared identity.

Thus, one may not see themselves as a palliative care provider but rather identify as a caregiver at work, at home, and at leisure.

Some consider callings through a religious lens while others link meaningful work to passion. Regardless, scholars agree that a calling is an important psychological state that emphasizes skill variety, task identity, and significance.

Benefits of Meaningful Work

- Increased occupational skill
- More autonomy
- Increased job satisfaction
- Enhanced work–life balance
- Feeling as though one is utilizing one's personal skills/talents to the fullest
- Giving back to the community

Considering the personal responsibility and challenges associated with emotional labor–intensive positions, many tend to associate these positions with a calling or meaningful work that actively contributes to individual well-being (see Box 7.1). According to one palliative care physician, "these human interaction experiences that we can have, not only do they drain—they can—but we receive a lot from them, and we get energized by the work that we do and the potential impact that you have. And I think that, in a sense, insulates from some of [the harmful effects of emotional labor]."

In a routine shift, a palliative care provider will engage in a variety of discussions and situations that require emotional work. This work is likely to emerge in the following communicative situations (e.g., Considine & Miller, 2010; Funk, Peters, & Roger, 2017; Vedel et al., 2014):

■ Helping patients and families to navigate confusion surrounding serious illness or end of life

■ Discussing care options in the absence of curative treatment

■ Providing patients with pain management strategies

■ Mitigating family dynamics

■ Engaging in conversations with patients and families about end-of-life, which may include religious, spiritual, or existential concerns

■ Assisting patients and their families in treatment and care decisions

■ Serving as the first line of bereavement when a patient dies

In addition to the emotion involved in the daily role responsibilities of palliative care, PCT members may experience emotional labor stemming from the personal grief that comes with caring for those with serious illnesses and at end of life (Funk et al., 2017). Thus, even though PCT members may feel as though they need to emote in specific ways (e.g., crying, yelling, taking a break), they are also expected to carry on as usual. This can help to exemplify why those "with an extra compassion bone" are often tagged for inclusion on PCTs and why Donald, a registered nurse in a pediatric palliative care unit, describes his ability to empathize as "his strongest trait and his kryptonite" (Omilion-Hodges & Swords, 2016, p. 331).

A Two-Pronged Approach to Emotional Labor

Emotional labor is commonly considered in two distinct veins: job-focused and employee-focused.

Job-focused emotional labor: This aspect of emotional labor relates to the frequency, intensity, and expectations associated with the performance of emotions on the job. Applied to palliative care, this may entail approaching each patient and family interaction as if it were the first appointment of the day—where PCT members enter each encounter with their undivided attention and with energy (Box 7.2). This can be a tall order considering the length of provider shifts, the frequency of patient appointments, and the intensity of topics tackled during patient–provider interactions. Taken together, job-focused emotional labor addresses interpersonal work demands, including the duration and frequency of interactions with patients and their families and emotion control, where PCT members are expected to emote in predictable

BOX 7.2

A NURSE REFLECTS: TREATING EACH PATIENT AS THE FIRST ONE OF THE DAY

It was just one of those days. There were these five ladies who'd survived cancer together for over five years that I knew well, and one of them died. And I saw one of the other group members and cried with her over the death. And then I dried my tears and took a deep breath and went to see my next patient who I've also known for a long time, and she's not going to make it. And I cried outside her room, and then I dried my tears, took a deep breath, and went to see my next patient.

ways (i.e., in treating each patient encounter with the same degree of attention, concern, and sincerity).

Employee-focused emotional labor: Whereas job-focused emotional labor relates to occupational expectations, employee-focused emotional labor is specific to each individual team member. This aspect of emotional labor details how individuals process and make sense of managing their emotions to fulfill their professional responsibilities. In palliative care contexts, employee-focused emotional labor seeks to answer the following question: How do healthcare professionals regulate and/or modify their emotions as they work to fulfill patient and other role-related needs? The extent to which healthcare professionals find emotional labor debilitating varies. For example, when discussing work–life balance, APRN Kalista shared that:

"I have those issues anyway. I bring those with me. The work doesn't really affect that … Part of that comes from my style of wanting to make my supervisor look good. Those are internally driven neuroses of work–life balance issues and I've had those at every job. The good thing about this team is that everybody here will remind me when that gets out of balance."

Two distinct processes are part and parcel with employee-focused emotional labor: *surface acting* and *deep acting*. Though it sounds less onerous than deep acting, surface acting can lead to negative outcomes for providers. Surface acting involves PCT members modifying their outward expressions and behaviors to hide their authentic feelings. While this can be as minor as putting on a smile to conceal a bad mood, over time surface acting can lead to serious physical and psychological concerns. Additionally, surface acting has been linked to three dimensions of burnout: emotional exhaustion, depersonalization, and diminished accomplishment (Brotheridge & Grandey, 2002). Kamal et al. (2016) found that of the 62% of palliative care professionals experiencing burn-out, most stemmed from emotional exhaustion with depersonalization serving as a minor component.

PCTs can serve as a protective factor against surface acting. While profession-al practice may require situations of hiding authentic feelings, teams are a place where such feelings can be shared. Since team members spend so much time with one another, they are also good observers of the possible signs of burnout. Sharing feelings and experiences with the team also allows for another type of processing—humor. While many outside of healthcare do not see anything hu-morous in death or serious illness, all jobs have funny moments and occurrences. The important thing is using the right lens, when appropriate, to find the humor or lightness in even the most trying of situations (see Boxes 7.3A and 7.3B).

BOX 7.3A

SOCIAL MEDIA AS SUPPORT: FINDING VALIDATION AND HUMOR IN TWEETS

In addition to sharing stories in person, team members may post to social media or share posts that they see with one another. For example, the Twitter feed Palliative Dork shares stories about "Geeking out about anything and everything in palliative care" but also shows organizational tensions with tweets like:

"Is it inappropriate to type 'I told you so' in a progress note?" (May 29, 2019)

"Palliative: Have had extensive, daily goals of care discussions, family requests more time to consider x5 days and counting. Geriatrics: Poor prognosis. Appreciate Palliative Medicine assistance—currently FULL CODE.–Yelling to get our attention? We KNOW." (April 5, 2019)

These social media posts display frustration that helps the palliative community feel connected and validated if they relate to the feelings. Another way to connect is through humor, and tweets often rely on humor that is specific to the field such as:

"Today I heard Miralax® mispronounced as Miracle-lax. I really don't think it produces poop miraculously, but I will call it this from now on." (May 22, 2019)

SOURCE: Palliative Dork [@PCDorkClub]. Tweets: 5/29/19, 5/14/19, 4/5/19. Retrieved from https://twitter.com/PCDorkClub

BOX 7.3B

HUMOR AT WORK: SOCIAL WORKER AND NURSE REFLECTIONS

A Social Worker Reflects

We do a lot of inappropriate humor. I think it is typical hospital humor. A lot of humor about dying that people might think is irreverent. But we know the boundaries of it. I mean—it would never get said, obviously, outside of this conference room, or outside of 4 East. But I think you have to laugh. And one of the things that I appreciate about this group is their sense of humor. We get to laughing so hard that it's ridiculous. And it's a huge release.

A Nurse Reflects

I think it helps. Humor is certainly one of our ways that we help with coping. And it also creates some of the team camaraderie stuff that goes on, too. You know? It's okay that you can laugh at yourself. I think that also levels the playing field for us that we can laugh at ourselves and just realize "This was really crazy" or "I can't believe this just happened to me." Just sharing your story helps.

Deep acting is a more emotionally complex phenomenon. Unlike surface acting where PCT members occasionally fake emotions to meet role demands, deep acting describes the internal processes team members experience as they work through their emotions and make sense of their feelings and actions related to their role. This can help to reduce the discomfort associated with having to remain cheerful or brave in trying situations because PCT members who engage in deep acting will set aside time to address these feelings. Thus, while they may not be able to cry on the unit after losing a special patient, it is likely that they will take time on a break or after shift's end to lean into those feelings. Considering that it is the most emotionally healthy route, deep acting has also been linked to meaningful work. In palliative care, PCT members may enact specific emotions not only because they feel mandated by the organization to do so, but also because of their sincere belief that all patients are deserving of genuine interactions (Box 7.4).

While the education of palliative care professionals includes information and even warnings about the signs of burnout, it can be difficult to see while it is happening. The cumulative nature of the emotional wear and tear of the job can erode a PCT member's sense of normative reactions. Even healthcare professionals who

BOX 7.4

A PALLIATIVE CARE PHYSICIAN REFLECTS ON EMOTIONAL LABOR AND MEANINGFUL WORK

Nurses and other human services workers report high levels of deep acting, which is related to a strong sense of personal fulfillment and a decrease in depersonalization (Brotheridge & Grandey, 2002). This finding also helps to illustrate the link between palliative care and meaningful work.

Allan, a palliative care physician on a high-performing palliative care team, finds that the work itself helps him to deal with the emotional labor associated with the role:

"I think there are some things that offset the draining portion of it, and part of it is just that, recognizing that 'We made a difference in this particular situation. This could have gone really bad,' or 'This was heading down a path.' And when you see that happening, even though it's very emotionally engaging, and you feel drained at times—you do—there is also this filling of the well again by your colleagues, as well as just the meaning of the work."

are more adept in general at deep acting and processing feelings associated with emotional work are not immune to compassion fatigue or burnout.

Compassion Satisfaction and Compassion Fatigue

Compassion is a core component of palliative care. In fact, many are drawn to palliative care and the field of medicine because of the joy that comes from helping others and the importance of working with patients and families as they experience serious illness.

Compassion Satisfaction

Compassion satisfaction stems from the positive feelings or validation that comes from being able to provide treatment (when applicable) and care to help alleviate pain and suffering in patients. In fact, compassion satisfaction is so integral to palliative care that it has been linked to (Sans et al., 2015):

- Provider quality of life
- Provider self-awareness
- Increased ability to cope with death
- A decreased likelihood of burnout

Part of compassion satisfaction is practicing awareness and integrating self-care practices into your daily routine. Practicing self-care individually and making it part of team practices can also help to prevent burnout, decrease team member conflict, guard against decreased empathy, and reduce absenteeism and turnover (Sans et al., 2015).

Compassion Fatigue

While compassion satisfaction is a contributor to higher work morale, compassion fatigue is the enemy of the helping professions. Compassion fatigue (Joinson, 1992) initially emerged in a study exploring burnout in emergency department nurses. In the face of extreme and continued tragedy, PCT members may lose their ability to form meaningful attachments with patients and to provide quality care. Recently, Cross (2019) further differentiated compassion fatigue from related concepts (e.g., burnout, secondary traumatic stress [STS], moral distress) in order to propose a definition specific to palliative care nursing. In this context, compassion fatigue is described as the condition that occurs when "compassion and empathy are lost, demonstrated by emotional and psychological, intellectual and professional, physical, social, and spiritual characteristics that, if left unattended, result in disinterest, moral distress, burnout, and breakdown" (Cross, 2019, p. 26).

Thus, compassion fatigue does not emerge solely from witnessing the pain and trauma of patients; it also emerges from heavy and/or expanding workloads, long shifts, or working within a culture that does not permit or promote opportunities for PCT members to talk about work-related stressors. PCT members are more vulnerable to compassion fatigue in certain circumstances including the following (Mooney et al., 2017; Sanchez-Reilly et al., 2013; Swetz, Harrington, Matsuyama, Shanafelt, & Lyckholm, 2009):

- Being new or early within your career
- Untenable environmental issues such as unsustainable workload, poor management, and limited or no opportunities for professional or personal development
- Being female
- Working in an intensive care unit
- Feeling as though work-related circumstances are out of your control

■   Attributing your successes to chance or external factors rather than reflecting on your own expertise and achievement

Teams that act more like a group of loosely connected individuals rather than as a true integrated interdisciplinary team may also contribute to provider compassion fatigue.

While considering these factors, it is important to remember that according to author Dr. Beth Hudnall Stamm, developer of the Professional Quality of Life (ProQOL) measure, "compassion fatigue is not a diagnosis. It is possible that compassion fatigue is a descriptive term and that a person struggling with compassion fatigue also has a psychological disorder" (https://proqol.org/CS _and_CF.html). For example, one PCT member may be experiencing compassion fatigue and also have a diagnosable level of depression. However, another PCT member may have compassion fatigue and not show signs of clinical depression.

While a number of different models of compassion fatigue exist, four components stand out as contributors to this phenomenon: burnout, secondary trauma, cumulative grief, and moral distress caused by feelings of helplessness (ProQOL; Sorenson, Bolick, Wright, & Hamilton, 2016). When a combination of these factors outweighs the feelings of compassion satisfaction, compassion fatigue may occur. Research also indicates prevalent compassion fatigue among counselors, social workers, and physicians—all key players in PCTs. Compassion fatigue is related to the following outcomes in palliative care professionals (Sans et al., 2015):

■   Increased likelihood of burnout
■   Decreased ability to cope with death
■   Decreases in self-awareness

Given the impact on individuals and teams, it is important to understand the elements and effects of compassion fatigue (Box 7.5 and Figure 7.1).

Burnout

Though the terms are not synonymous, *compassion fatigue* and *burnout* are often used interchangeably when discussing emotional labor positions. In the context of palliative care, burnout has been described as feelings of helplessness over one's work environment and the ability to make a difference (Cross, 2019). Burnout also tends to occur over a longer period of time (Sorenson et al., 2016). Further, Boyle (2011) pointed out that there are three distinguishing

BOX 7.5

COMPASSION FATIGUE IN PALLIATIVE CARE TEAM MEMBERS

In addition to feeling as though they are unable to emotionally connect with patients and role responsibilities, team members experiencing compassion fatigue may also experience (Boyle, 2011):

- The inability to sleep or, conversely, the desire to stay in bed
- Headaches
- Moodiness
- Gastrointestinal distress

PCT members experiencing compassion fatigue report feeling ineffective at work because of a looming feeling of apathy or the inability to nurture others.

Potential Lasting Effects

If left untreated, compassion fatigue may permanently alter a provider's ability to enact compassionate care and finding meaning in role responsibilities (Boyle, 2011).

Compassion Fatigue Is Progressive

If PCT members do not take steps to seek professional help, find social support, and begin integrating self-care practices, they may not be able to return to experiencing the compassion satisfaction and the meaningful work they once knew.

---

factors between burnout and compassion fatigue: causes, timing, and outcomes (addressed in Exhibit 7.1).

Burnout for Underresourced Palliative Care Staff

While the differences between burnout and compassion fatigue are spelled out in Exhibit 7.1, it is important to note that palliative care members also have a high propensity for burnout. Over 50% of palliative care physicians are predicted to leave the practice by 2024 (Cavallo, 2014). Part of the reason that burnout is as prevalent as it is for palliative care providers is that patient demand often exceeds staffing (O'Connor, 2018). The perception of work as meaningful can be protective of burnout. However, as a study by Shanafelt et al. (2009) found, that protection has a limit. The researchers found that "those spending less than 20% of their time on the activity that is most meaningful to them had higher rates of burnout—53.8% vs. 29.9%" (p. 990).

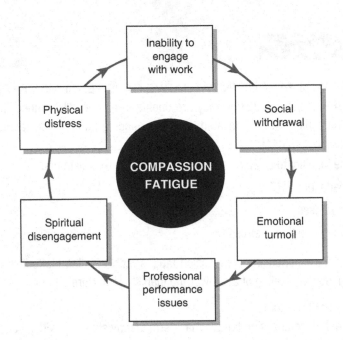

FIGURE 7.1 Outcomes of compassion fatigue.

EXHIBIT 7.1

DISTINGUISHING BETWEEN COMPASSION FATIGUE AND BURNOUT

1. Causes: What may prompt burnout or compassion fatigue?

Burnout—Linked to traditional organizational stressors such as heavy workloads, limited or inadequate personnel, material, or financial resources, and poor or trying leader–member or peer relationships.

Compassion fatigue—While burnout is linked to team member reactions to the work environment, compassion fatigue is linked to the relational strain found in emotional labor–intensive positions.

2. Timing: When does burnout or compassion fatigue set in?

Burnout—Because burnout is linked with environmental issues such as increased workload and/or deteriorating peer or leader–member relationships, it tends to emerge slowly over time.

Compassion fatigue—In contrast to burnout, compassion fatigue tends to be emergent. That is, after a particularly trying case, clinicians may find themselves feeling as though they do not even recognize themselves, their feelings, or their behaviors.

3. Outcomes: How does burnout or compassion fatigue manifest or present in healthcare professionals?

Burnout—Many times those who are experiencing burnout transfer to different units or teams or different organizations. This is because the root of the discomfort is not related to the occupation, but rather the specific unit, team, or organization.

Compassion fatigue—Those experiencing compassion fatigue will often try to bear the imbalance between administering treatment and the loss of empathy. If left untreated or if these feelings do not abate, healthcare providers may leave the occupation or attempt to start over in a new organization.

As palliative care professionals and teams are susceptible to burnout, creating and adhering to a team strategy for managing common work stressors may prove helpful. The PCT at the Hospital of the University of Pennsylvania serves as an excellent example. The team routinely found itself facing a daily census that exceeded the staff's ability to provide high-quality care. Instead of continuing to overstretch their limited resources, they strategized workflow practices for managing their growing consult demand (O'Connor, 2018):

1. Prioritize consults who are most likely to benefit from palliative care. That is, some consults may be better served by others (e.g., psychiatric social worker or pain management team) rather than the PCT.

2. Establish program-wide criteria to help decide which consults should continue with palliative care for the long term and which cases are able to be signed off on.

3. Determine if an interdisciplinary approach is required for the case—not every consult requires one. Members of this PCT consider the specifics of each case and determine if a social worker or a pharmacist, for example, may be better equipped than a physician or advanced practice provider (APP) to handle a consult.

4. Hold office hours with or regularly visit key referral sources to provide informational education and triage and streamline incoming consults.

5. Implement a cap. While this may not feel like an ideal solution, when consults vastly exceed staffing, it may be the only option. This approach should be discussed with organizational leadership and may serve to illustrate the need for additional resources.

Being an underresourced PCT is stressful. Exhibit 7.2 highlights a conversation between team members where one member needs to vent and the other member assists her in remembering why she continues to do this work. Kelsey demonstrates active listening while also helping her colleague to reframe her situation. Since they have had this conversation many times before, Kelsey knows this is what Lillian needs right now—validation that her feelings of frustration are legitimate and a reminder that there are job perks here that she might not find elsewhere.

EXHIBIT 7.2

TALKING THROUGH MOMENTS OF STRESS

Whenever Lillian, an RN, has a tough day, she tends to have the following conversation with Kelsey, a social worker. While it is a repetitive conversation, it seems to be one that helps Lillian reframe her work and situation each time.

Lillian: I don't know why I even do this work! RNs aren't paid anything. I should just quit and do something else.

Kelsey: Well, you know you could. Although, it might be a hassle to look for a job.

Lillian: Yeah, it would.

Kelsey: But you might make more money somewhere else.

Lillian: I'd probably make a lot more.

Kelsey: Hmmm ... I wonder who you would work with?

Lillian: I wouldn't have the people I have here.

Kelsey: This is benefits versus burdens. No different than we do when we try to help our patients. Like, this location isn't convenient for me and I know I'm paid less than some other social workers. But this team, this team is a gift.

Lillian: Yeah, this team is a gift.

Secondary Traumatic Stress

Working in palliative care can be stressful, even traumatic, at times. Providers who are personally involved in a traumatic event may experience primary traumatic stress. For example, a nurse who fractures a frail, elderly patient's ribs while performing CPR may experience this phenomenon. The feelings associated with primary traumatic stress may last for a long time even with appropriate coping techniques, a good support system, and possibly professional counseling.

While primary trauma is easier to identify as an occupational stressor, secondary traumatic stress, also known as vicarious trauma, is an underacknowledged factor in compassion fatigue (Sorenson et al., 2016). Given the nature of palliative care work, professionals in this field are closely involved with patients and families experiencing tragic or painful events. If secondary traumatic stress is not acknowledged and addressed, palliative care professionals' morale may begin to erode.

Cumulative Grief

Cumulative grief is another contributor to compassion fatigue (Carton & Hupcey, 2014; Spilman, 2010). Constant exposure to sorrow, suffering, and death is a reality for PCT members. Additionally, PCT members are not necessarily afforded time to grieve for each patient before there is another loss. Spilman (2010) acknowledges that feelings of loss can be even greater if the members feel as though they were unable to provide a patient with a good death. Because cumulative grief is linked to compassion fatigue and burnout, research such as Carton and Hupcey (2014) reiterates the need to establish effective procedures that allow PCT members to adequately address the loss of their patients. For example, PCTs may use rituals (Box 7.6) to mark the deaths of patients and consider the meaning of their work as a part of those patients' and families' experiences.

Moral Distress and Feelings of Helplessness

Moral distress in palliative care may be the result of the inability to reconcile professional integrity with the clinical care situation. In other words, it is the feeling that something that is not good for the patient is happening anyway and the provider feels helpless to do anything about it. Palliative care professionals may experience moral distress as follows:

BOX 7.6

A CHAPLAIN REFLECTS: ACKNOWLEDGING THE DEATH OF PATIENTS THROUGH RITUAL

Once a month, we use part of our weekly team meeting to acknowledge the passing of our patients. We have a basket of stones and a glass bowl. During the monthly ritual, we pick up a stone from the basket, say the patient's name, and place the stone into the bowl. As the stone is transferred, we might share something about the patient or our experiences with this person or family. No one is required to speak, and the stone might pass silently to the bowl—it's a space for people to speak up if they want to. After all of the names are spoken aloud, a chaplain offers a blessing. Every few months, once the basket is empty, we pass the bowl around from person to person. While we pass the bowl, we take a moment and appreciate the weight of the stones in the bowl. We think about how we experience that cumulative weight as palliative care professionals. Then we return the stones to the basket.

- Medical Futility: "Why would cardiology even offer that? They know it isn't going to help, and they just don't want to tell the patient."
- Injustice: "The system is broken! This medication would help the patient, but their insurance won't cover it. They expect the patient to pay out of pocket, and this person just can't."
- Colleagues' Choices: "That's not how to talk to this family. I know it isn't my job to tell a colleague how to act, but now the family doesn't trust us anymore. I don't think we have enough time left with this patient to rebuild that trust and help them like we do best."

All of the preceding examples involve feelings of helplessness on the part of the provider. When your vocation is patient care and the ability to best care for the patient is compromised by factors outside of your control, you may experience feelings of helplessness. These feelings may also be labeled as moral distress. PCT members will all likely experience feelings of helplessness throughout their careers due to the nature of the work (Back, Rushton, Kaszniak, & Halifax, 2015; Cavallo, 2014).

Some have suggested using the feeling of helplessness as a barometer for gauging one's level of engagement with patients at any given time (Back et al., 2015). The researchers suggest that just as you would not expect a barometer to be static, it is not reasonable to expect that a PCT member's levels of empathy and engagement will be either. Illness progression can be unpredictable by nature, which, in turn, means that patients, their families, and PCT members may often feel like they are on an emotional rollercoaster. Back et al. (2015) suggest that this may lead members to experience a variety of sweeping emotions from apathy (hypo-engagement) to anxiety and extreme vigilance (hyperengagement).

One way to address feelings of helplessness and the related challenges are to RENEW (Recognize, Embrace, Nourish, Embody, Weave). In their RENEW model, Back et al. (2015, p. 28) reiterate the importance for PCT members to (Figure 7.2):

1. Recognize: Take the time to recognize when feelings of helplessness are present

2. Embrace: Lean into their mental and physical feelings and address them (i.e., recognizing that you need time to process is not the same as taking time to process a case)

3. Nourish: Engage in nourishing or self-care behaviors that help them to feel restored

4. Embody: Enact engagement in terms of reconnecting with the challenging case or situation. This may include deep breathing or other mindfulness activities (refer to Boxes 7.10, 7.16, and 7.17 for examples specific to palliative care)

5. Weave: Select a new response that is both emotionally and cognitively healthy for them as caregivers

Box 7.7 highlights additional practical steps implemented by a high-performing PCT in order to continue to deliver exemplary patient-centered care while also helping to protect PCT members' well-being.

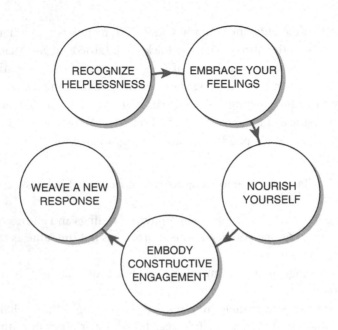

FIGURE 7.2 RENEW Model: Consider how to renew when feelings of helplessness present.

SOURCE: From Back, A. L., Rushton, C. H., Kaszniak, A. W., & Halifax, J. S. (2015). "Why are we doing this?": Clinician helplessness in the face of suffering. *Journal of Palliative Medicine, 18*(1), 26–30. doi:10.1089/jpm.2014.0115

BOX 7.7

PRACTICAL WORKFLOW STRATEGIES FOR OVERWORKED PALLIATIVE CARE PROGRAMS

One high-performing palliative care team integrated the following practical strategies to manage their growing referral volume:

1. Hired and trained prn staff (social worker, chaplain, APRN) to work during high census periods and to cover other members when they are on leave or on vacation

2. Hired an additional APRN for both inpatient and outpatient service expansion

3. Developed intentional and consensus-based processes for signing off when no unmet specialty-level palliative care needs are identified

4. Developed a palliative care acuity system to facilitate appropriate "dosing" of palliative care professionals

5. Re-engaged team members in role delineation activities based on palliative care domains to ensure respect for professional roles and avoidance of task overlap

6. Designed streamlined note templates to improve efficiency while maintaining excellent communication and documentation standards

7. Acquired new office space to accommodate new hires and allow for close interdisciplinary collaboration throughout the workday

8. Created primary palliative care training strategies for nonspecialty staff

9. Engaged available services from an administrative assistant to take on chart review/data entry tasks from the RN coordinator

10. Developed a volunteer bereavement card coordinator position to relieve chaplains from an administrative task

11. Implemented team-building and self-care strategies to prevent burnout

Compassion fatigue and its components saddle healthcare professionals and interdisciplinary care teams with additional emotional burdens to bear and weather. Moreover, each requires immediate and sustained attention in addition to a re-evaluation of work–life balance and integration of self-care practices. As Faith, a director of palliative care, describes palliative care work: "It's messy, it's sad, it's a heartbreakingly real time for our patients. We can't appear, even for a moment, that we don't care, that we're not standing right there beside them" (Omilion-Hodges & Swords, 2016, p. 332). There is a lot at stake—the care of the patient and family, as well as the ability of the provider to continue to do the job well and to be a functioning part of an interdisciplinary team. Therefore, paying attention to the causes of compassion fatigue and working to ensure a robust sense of compassion satisfaction are important.

It is one thing to notice the signs of compassion fatigue and another thing to do something about it at the team and/or organizational level. It would seem the simplest solution is encouraging team members to pass patients to another healthcare professional when compassion fatigue or its components are recognized. However, the use of this simple solution requires healthy teams who have a high degree of trust in one another and a willingness to encourage members to express when they are feeling overwhelmed. Team or organizational solutions

BOX 7.8

CALLING A CODE LAVENDER

Code Lavender began as a crisis intervention tool at a Hawaiian hospital in 2004. A healthcare professional calling this code is signaling that he or she is having a rough time at work. When the code is called, the struggling team member receives a small packet of items. A study at the University of California San Diego teaching hospital distributed packets containing a lavender aromatherapy vial, a piece of chocolate, and a handwritten note with an encouraging quote. In this study, 100% of those receiving the packet found it to be helpful. While it did not change their Professional Quality of Life posttest scores, participants did report feeling that the organization recognized them and cared for them (Davidson et al., 2017).

such as Code Lavender (see Box 7.8) can be effective if the participants believe that letting others know they are feeling burnout will result in support. Mechanisms like this can be a boon to individual and team morale, but it is also important to note that team-care solutions such as passing off patients and Code Lavenders will not make up for underresourced teams over the long term. Finally, even in teams with great team-care practices, it is also important for individual PCT members to practice self-care.

What Is Self-Care?

Self-care is an essential component of personal and emotional well-being. Self-care encompasses routine opportunities and integrated moments of care designed for balance, nourishment, and renewal. The Hospice and Palliative Medicine subspecialty identifies self-care as integral to provider well-being, satisfaction, and career longevity. In fact, the 2018 Annual Assembly of Hospice and Palliative Care held a town hall meeting dedicated to discussing the importance of clinician well-being and resilience by stressing the importance of self-care (Dahlin, Mastrojohn, & Rotella, 2018).

It is important to note that self-care is *not*:

- A new-agey fad
- Indulgent

- A luxury
- Expensive
- Time intensive
- Optional

Self-care can be integrated into any schedule and any budget. Acts of self-care can help you to recharge and to maintain harmony between your occupational role and your personal roles (e.g., parent, spouse, friend, neighbor, community member; Box 7.9). Moreover, self-care is just as important for your physical health as it is for your mental well-being. Self-care also directly affects PCT members' quality of life. Compared with their peers who do not routinely engage in self-care, professionals who enact self-care practices enjoy a higher quality of life in addition to reporting higher levels of resilience and overall wellness (Ayala, Winseman, Johnsen, & Mason, 2018; Melvin, 2015; Omilion-Hodges & Swords, 2016; Sans et al., 2015).

BOX 7.9

A PHYSICIAN REFLECTS: THE CRAP-TO-FUN RATIO

When I've approached burnout, it's because I have not had enough time to have diversions. One of the things I came across when I was in college was the idea of rotating crops. Having things in your life that replenish you in different ways is helpful. I'm comfortable going from one activity to the next and trying to stay engaged realizing "Each one of these has different ways of replenishing you and filling your bucket." We have many dimensions to ourselves as human beings, and we have to touch all of those and try to build them into our life experience. Physically? I exercise. Spiritually? We go to church as a family, and I do daily practice for myself. Socially? As a physician, I'm in contact with people all the time and I really enjoy what I do. I also get to teach and sometimes play an administrative role. I tell people "You know, there's crap in our life and there's fun in our life. You have to manage the crap-to-fun ratio in your life. If there's too much crap, you have to go look for the fun, for the part you enjoy."

Recent research (Ayala, Omorodion, Nmecha, Winseman, & Mason, 2017) identified clusters of self-care activities reported by medical students (see Box 7.10).

BOX 7.10

SELF-CARE ACTIVITIES FOR HEALTHCARE PROFESSIONALS
Researchers (Ayala et al., 2017) identified 10 clusters of self-care activities as reported by medical students:

1. **Nourishment:** Eating healthfully, staying hydrated

2. **Hygiene:** Maintain physical health and appearance, getting adequate sleep, pampering (e.g., baths, long showers, manicures)

3. **Intellectual and creative health:** Follow current events; enjoy books and podcasts, and creative activities (knitting, choir, instruments, photography)

4. **Physical activity:** Regular exercise

5. **Spiritual care:** Attend religious services, pray, meditate, journal, reflection, therapy

6. **Balance and relaxation:** Designated downtime, boundaries, taking time off, breathing exercises

7. **Time for loved ones:** Dedicated time with romantic partners, family, and friends

8. **Big picture goals:** Consider 5- and 10-year plans

9. **Pleasure and outside activities:** Dinner out, time outdoors, cooking

10. **Hobbies:** Writing, reading for pleasure, arts and crafts, recreational sports

SOURCE: Ayala, E. E., Omorodion, A. M., Nmecha, D., Winseman, J. S., & Mason, H. R. C. (2017). What do medical students do for self-care? A student-centered approach to well-being. *Teaching and Learning in Medicine: An International Journal, 29*(3), 237–246. doi:10.1080/10401334.2016 .1271334

Benefits of Self-Care

Self-care offers individuals a wealth of positive outcomes. In addition to being linked to increases in PCT members' quality of life, engaging in self-care practices can also result in the following benefits:

■ **Work–Life Balance:** While many palliative care professionals find meaning and fulfillment in their work, it does not mean the role should be all consuming. Integrating self-care allows PCT members to enjoy a balanced life where they find enjoyment in work and non–work-related activities (Box 7.9).

■ **Stress Management:** Self-care is an effective means of addressing and alleviating stress. In addition to exercise, meditation, journaling, and prayer are commonly cited sources of stress abatement (Ayala et al., 2017).

- **Personal Worth:** While many palliative care professionals identify as caregivers in and out of the clinical environment, they should practice turning those self-nurturing skills inward as well. The idea is reminiscent of the airline instructions to put on your mask before assisting others with theirs. In order to help patients, you must be healthy enough to be helpful. It is important to remember that neglecting self-care is not noble and is likely to result in feeling overwhelmed, stressed, and distracted in all facets of life including patient care.

- **Physical Health:** Without physical health, PCT members cannot care for their patients, their families, or themselves. Maintaining physical health can include engaging in regular physical activity, eating well, staying hydrated, and getting 7–9 hours of sleep as recommended by the National Sleep Foundation (2015). It is also important to make time for routine health checkups in addition to seeing experts for additional physical, mental, or emotional maintenance or concerns.

Self-Care Is Essential

In times of stress, such as high patient census or when teams are understaffed, PCT members' initial reaction may be to skip a break or put off lunch as a way to accomplish more work. They may cancel evening plans with friends or skip their regular Pilates class so that they can stay late to work on patient charts. Unfortunately, while this is a common practice, it is not a healthy one. Self-care is always important, but it becomes even more so as stress ramps up. Additionally, while cancelling plans and missing an occasional lunch break are not causes for concern if done rarely, these actions may have larger ramifications if done frequently. Most palliative care professionals know what would be a good self-care regimen but fail to follow through. As there is a link between commitment and consistency (Cialdini, 2009), taking the time to set goals and creating a plan to realize those goals increases the chance of follow-through.

Balancing Your Needs in a Team Context

Palliative care is hard but essential work. The impact of work-related stress on PCT members' well-being has long been documented (Berman, Campbell, Makin, & Todd, 2007; Kearney, Weininger, Vachon, Harrison, & Mount, 2009; Martins Pereira, Fonseca, & Sofia Carvalho, 2011). PCTs (not just individual practitioners) are also susceptible to occupational stressors, which can lead to breakdowns in communication, provider withdrawal, and medical errors (Sanchez-Reilly et al., 2013; West et al., 2006). This prompts two natural questions:

1. How do palliative care professionals balance their individual needs within the team context?
2. What can teams do to integrate self-care and team care into their daily roles and team processes?

The first question is explored in this section, and the chapter concludes with team-level suggestions for enhancing resiliency and decreasing stress while delivering intentional patient-centered care. While palliative care professionals can develop a solid foundation of wellness and resiliency through the personal self-care activities (e.g., exercise, meditation, spending time with friends and family), there are also workplace-specific actions that can help to create a barrier against burnout and compassion fatigue.

In a thorough review of self-care activities related to palliative care professionals and oncologists, Sanchez-Reilly et al. (2013) suggest that providers engage in the following organizational activities:

- Developing and maintaining strong peer relationships
- Seeking out mentors
- Finding new ways to engage within the organization
- Reflecting regularly on workplace performance
- Improving management and communication skills
- Practicing mindfulness at work (Box 7.11)

BOX 7.11

A CHAPLAIN REFLECTS: LEADING A BREATHING EXERCISE AT THE BEGINNING OF ROUNDS EACH MORNING

I make them breathe every morning because it is important for us to just take the time and center ourselves—particularly for what we are dealing with. If I can just get them to inhale and exhale, it's good for each of us. When I first suggested it, they thought it was nice. But they thought it was just going to be that one time! And then the next day, they were ready to jump into patient care, and I said "Well, are we gonna breathe?" Some people are a little high strung and anxious some days, but I'm thinking "All I ask you for is 2 minutes of your time—2 minutes when I could ask you for 5 or 10." But I don't do that. And I wouldn't get it if I did. Now whoever is leading the meeting prompts me to start the breathing while also saying "And then we'll start on…" To me, that's acceptance versus "I hope she doesn't start with the breathing!"

These suggestions largely align with the primary dimensions of self-care: physical, emotional, spiritual, financial, social, workplace, and future goal setting. Social integration, for example, gives PCT members sources of social support. Thus, rather than looking at the development of peer relationships as frivolous, recognizing the power of connecting with others who understand the unique highs and lows of palliative care is priceless and may offer the following benefits:

- Processing difficult emotions with others who have an intimate understanding of specific cases
- Having trusted confidants in the workplace (which may develop into lasting friendships)
- Access to work-related advice (e.g., pain or symptom management, how to deal with the team leader)
- Access to job-related affirmation for your skills and decision-making
- A barrier against isolation

Many suggestions (Sanchez-Reilly et al., 2013) for individual self-care within organizational settings align with the emotional and professional health and future goal-setting dimensions of self-care.

- Self-care is not only about nourishing yourself now; it is also considering what steps or factors will allow you to continue to grow personally and professionally. Seeking mentors and finding new ways to engage at work are clear paths for doing so.
- Taking time to reflect on work performance can enhance your emotional and professional health. This allows you to consider areas for improvement, additional skills, or training you would like to hone or acquire and consider how you see yourself developing as your career progresses. This reflection is also helpful in allowing palliative care professionals to consider if they have an interest in becoming a team leader or member of management in the future or if they would find more fulfillment in continued patient work.
- Practicing mindfulness in the workplace comes with a slew of benefits from increased patient-centered care, provider self-care and well-being, and development of enhanced empathy (Beckman et al., 2012; Kabat-Zinn, 2006; Mehta et al., 2016).
- Embracing empathy is another recommended way for palliative care professionals to deal with work-related stress (Harrison & Westwood, 2009; Kearney et al., 2009).

Protecting Oneself Through Empathy and Boundary Setting

A common misconception of displaying empathy, or engaging with and sharing feelings with another, is that it always depletes or takes away from a caregiver's personal well-being. However, Harrison and Westwood (2009) found that peer-nominated master therapists, including those in palliative care, used exquisite empathy to protect themselves from burnout and emotional depletion in addition to using traditional self-care measures such as seeking social support, practicing mindfulness, setting and maintaining boundaries (Box 7.12), and professional satisfaction and meaning.

BOX 7.12

UNINTENDED CONSEQUENCES OF SKIPPING LUNCH AND STAYING LATE

While it may feel like the only way to stay afloat is to skip breaks or to cancel plans to catch up, these actions come with unintended consequences. If you or one of your colleagues routinely engages in these behaviors, consider the associated outcomes and personal costs before doing so.

■ **You will not change the organization:** If your team is still able to care for patients and administrative needs are met, senior leadership may not be able to see the extent to which more resources are needed.

■ **You give your consent:** You tacitly okay this level of work and working conditions by consistently working through breaks or staying late or coming in early.

■ **You damage relationships:** Loved ones understand when you have to cancel occasionally—especially if it means that you take time to recharge your batteries and engage in self-care. However, if you repeatedly prioritize work over them, relationships may become strained.

■ **You deprive your physical and emotional well-being:** It is incredibly challenging to care for others if you are not properly caring for or addressing your own physical, emotional, and relational needs.

■ **You are too tired to provide exemplary care:** Sustained periods of stress including being understaffed, overworked, or picking up extra shifts can leave you unable to be the care provider you strive to be.

Exquisite empathy involves clarity about personal and interpersonal boundaries so that as PCT members develop meaningful connections with patients, they are also able to protect themselves from absorbing or taking on vicarious trauma (Harrison & Westwood, 2009). In this sense, connecting with the intent to create a collaborative, genuine alliance can actually contribute to PCT members' health through the meaning they find in the work. Put simply, leaning into natural feelings of compassion and embracing connections with patients may be more beneficial to PCT members than working to create distance or maintain very strict or rigid boundaries (Box 7.13).

BOX 7.13

PALLIATIVE CARE TEAM MEMBERS REFLECT ON THE NOURISHING POWER OF EMPATHY

John, a palliative care clinician in a faith-based health system: "I feel much closer to my patients and fuller as a person when they express their frustration, disappointment or fear and I'm able to look them in the eye and tell them 'I'm scared too' or 'I'm sad too.' They know that I'm there with them and I'm honoring myself, too, instead of pretending it's all okay or business as usual" (Omilion-Hodges & Swords, 2016, p. 332).

Warun, another palliative care physician from a high-performing team, also considers how empathetic encounters can enhance or contribute to provider well-being by reiterating the meaning of the work, saying:

"When you have some positive experiences—everybody's maybe a little bit different, but for me, one of the things that probably helps me through some of this is when you realize you've made a connection with the family and the patient, and you see the transformation occur during your encounter. You see that maybe you've been able to help with a catharsis, and you get people emoting better, and it's out there on the table, and you see that they're relieved at the end. You realize, 'That was good; that helped; that was an important piece.'"

How to Build Continual Self-Care and Team-Care Into Effective Teams

Just as PCT members are vulnerable to burnout, so are the teams themselves. This is especially true if environmental issues in the workplace, such as an unsustainable workload or poor management, continue to hamper a PCT's ability to focus on patient care.

This section builds on the previous with best practices and ideas that PCTs can integrate into their daily practices to protect themselves from some of the challenges of their occupation. Team leaders, in particular, may find these ideas helpful for facilitating a healthy work environment for team members by focusing on skills-based interventions that build resiliency (Back, Steinhauser, Kamal, & Jackson, 2016).

Figure 7.3 illustrates the most common factors that can contribute to a PCT's collective functioning through the development of strong leader and peer relationships, a sustainable workplace, and environment that is conducive to and rewarding of exemplary patient care.

1. **Environmental Factors:** High-stress and emotional labor–intensive work environments such as palliative care programs can be breeding grounds for burnout if not thoughtfully designed and run. Environmental factors, such as adequate work space, equipment, and staffing, can either help to foster a healthy environment that is conducive to patient-centered care or one that overburdens PCT members so that they are not able to focus primarily on

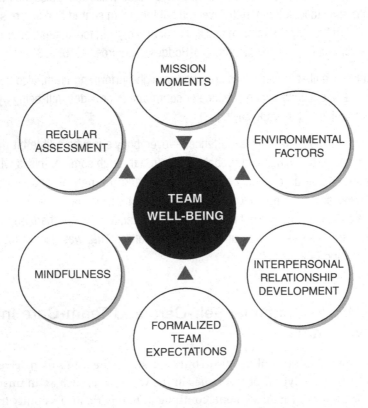

FIGURE 7.3 Factors that enhance team well-being and collective functioning.

patient needs. The importance of team leadership to mitigate these factors was discussed in Chapter 4, Leading Palliative Care Teams.

2. **Interpersonal Relationship Development:** One of the major strengths of palliative care—delivered via interdisciplinary teams—can also be a weakness if not approached thoughtfully. Members should be trained and spend time discussing individual and group roles. Team leaders can remind members of role flexing (Dahlin, Coyne, Goldberg, & Vaughan, 2019; Nancarrow et al., 2013) and blurring (Sims, Hewitt, & Harris, 2015) so that all members approach care from a perspective of "we" rather than "I." Studies recommend PCTs undergo training on group communication as a means to foster a supportive work community (Sanchez-Reilly et al., 2013; Shanafelt et al., 2005; Swetz et al., 2009). Similarly, team leaders should carve out time for members to enjoy some time socially together. This could be in the form of bringing in coffee and bagels before a meeting or catering a team lunch or another way for team members to spend some informal time together. Far from being seen as idle chatter, research shows that when team members get to know each other as people they are more likely to develop supportive, trusting two-way relationships (Omilion-Hodges & Ackerman, 2018). This is particularly important in the palliative care environment where members need to trust each other to augment and occasionally fill their own roles (see the example in Box 7.14).

BOX 7.14

SUPPORTIVE TEAM RELATIONSHIPS IN PALLIATIVE CARE

Johnny, a social worker in a palliative care program, shared an example of the importance peers can play in managing the emotions associated with palliative care. When he was the only social worker left on the team at 4:00 p.m. on Friday, Hadley, a palliative care clinical nurse specialist, came in and said "What can I do? I know you've had a rough day, and how can I help?" In addition to offering him assistance, Hadley also came bearing chocolate. While it was a minor gesture and one that may be seen as tangential to Hadley's own nursing responsibilities, Johnny reiterated how much the support meant: "…when we get distressed about a case, or upset, there's a lot of immediate support." This immediate support can help to assuage the negative effects of surface acting.

3. **Formalized Team Expectations:** Formalized team expectations largely stem from the team leader's explicit instructions and behaviors. A team leader, for example, may assign or encourage mentorship or work buddies. The former is often considered to be a more formal arrangement, where the mentor and mentee have regularly scheduled meetings, set collaborative

goals, and consider professional and personal indicators of success (Disch, 2018). The latter, while less formal, can pair professionals to create a first-line source of informational support in the form of job-related duties and of social support during especially trying days. Relatedly, team leaders should also articulate and uphold clear guidelines for addressing conflict and mis-communication among members (Box 7.15).

BOX 7.15

ACHIEVING A BETTER WORK DAY THROUGH FLEXIBILITY

One high-performing palliative care team noticed that, despite their best efforts to divvy up work evenly among PCT members in the morning, individual team members' responsibilities might take more or less time than expected. One PCT member might end up with a number of time-consuming events such as an unplanned family meeting, a patient death, or a new, complicated referral whereas another PCT member's day goes smoothly.

Rather than just sticking with the original plan for the day, which would leave the first PCT member to work late, a PCT leader suggested sending out a group text to the team at 2:30 p.m. to see who had capacity to take on some tasks to even out the work load a bit. They tried it for a week to evaluate its effect. Once they tweaked the intervention (changed the time to 3:00 p.m. and reassigned texting responsibility to the RN), they found that team members felt better supported and were more likely to leave work on time so they continued the practice.

For example, a team leader may notice an increase in chatter about an unsatisfactory interaction with a PCT member that does not include that person in the conversation. While venting can be healthy, this kind of talking about rather than with someone is not healthy for the team. Talking with the team member will also illuminate if the issue is a misunderstand-ing or a true conflict of interest or value. It is important that team leaders acknowledge that misunderstandings happen and often emerge because PCT members are steadfast in their commitment to patient care. In turn, team leaders must also formalize the steps that members, including the team leader, are expected to take if they need to resolve an issue or air a complaint with a peer.

4. **Mindfulness:** Aside from environmental factors, making PCT members aware of mindfulness and making space for the practice is likely the most impactful team factor for team and member wellness and well-being. Mind-fulness is the state of remaining present and focused in the moment. Such attentiveness is linked with adaptive, genuine, and reflective communication

(Burgoon, Berger, & Waldron, 2000). Practicing mindfulness and mindful communication in the healthcare environment has been linked to increased patient safety and delegation (Anthony & Vidal, 2010), provider and team wellness (Beckman et al., 2012; Mehta et al., 2016), and the ability to develop authentic relationships with patients (Omilion-Hodges & Swords, 2016).

An additional benefit of mindfulness is the many paths that lead to it (Box 7.16). For example, some PCTs have undergone stress reduction and mindfulness sessions collaboratively in order to build collective resiliency (Mehta et al., 2016), whereas individual practitioners may find that journaling, blogging, praying, or meditating will also help them to learn how to remain in the present (Kearney et al., 2009; Omilion-Hodges & Swords, 2016).

BOX 7.16

PREPARING FOR WORK, TACKLING THE DAY, AND LEAVING WORK AT WORK

Palliative care professionals have found that establishing routines for getting into the mind-set of work, remaining present at work, and preparing to transition home have been helpful. Here are some practices that you may also find helpful (drawn from Omilion-Hodges & Swords, 2016, p. 332).

Before work

■ Reflect on a personal care mantra (e.g., "I serve body, mind, and spirit").

At work

■ Using a pin, necklace, or other accessory as a reminder to stay present. One palliative care clinician wears a religious pin on her lab coat and touches it to remember to stay "in the present and attend fully to the patient."

After work

■ Journal or blog to reflect on the day before leaving for home in order to "reflect on the sanctity of my job" and "to process the emotions of the day."

Anytime

■ Mediation, prayer, and/or deep breathing to stay in the moment and practice mindfulness as a means to "remind us why we do this [palliative care]."

SOURCE: Omilion-Hodges, L. M., & Swords, N. M. (2016). Communication that heals: Mindful communication practices from palliative care leaders. *Health Communication, 31*(3), 328–335. doi:10.1080/10410236.2014.953739

5. **Regular Assessment:** Regular assessment allows the team leader and members to check in with their professional progress. This team-based factor involves having clearly defined processes and opportunities for professional development whether through continued medical education courses or by setting a tentative promotion plan with the team leader. Regular assessment also rests on honoring PCT members' autonomy to use their expertise as they see fit and rewarding those who continually demonstrate excellence in team-based patient-centered care (Balch & Copeland, 2007).

6. **Mission Moments:** In many ways, palliative care is mission work. That is, the focus of palliative care aligns with many healthcare centers' mission of providing holistic care. One clear way to boost and maintain team morale is to highlight the meaning of the work that is carried out by PCTs (Mehta et al., 2016). Team leaders may connect with their organization's marketing team to learn how to highlight members' contributions, and less formally, team leaders may consider awarding a weekly or monthly mission moment member by praising specific instances of exemplary care (Sanchez-Reilly et al., 2013). As Gus, a palliative care physician, explains, "I think the other piece that's part of it is that everybody generally enjoys their work, and that helps a lot. This is not drudgery at all." This aligns with suggestions (Harrison & Westwood, 2009) that drawing meaning from emotional labor–intensive positions and encouraging satisfaction in professional endeavors may help to protect members from burnout.

Keys to Integrating Self-Care Practices Into the Team Environment

Drawing from a successful PCT-based intervention designed to increase resiliency and decrease stress (Back et al., 2016; Mehta et al., 2016), three factors are likely to help facilitate self-care practices within the workplace.

1. **Palliative Care Professionals Must Be Involved From the Start:** Successful programs should be developed by or at least in concert with palliative care leaders and team members. Since they will ultimately be the end users of the practices or the self-care program, it is important that palliative care professionals are able to express needs and provide feedback in order to design interventions that directly apply to the work they do.

2. **Needs and Outcomes Should Be Clearly Identified:** In order for a new program or process to work, a clear need or gap must first be identified. PCTs may designate meeting time to prioritize self-care needs or

environmental issues that can be addressed that will decrease the collective stress of the program.

3. **Take a Skills-Based Approach:** By creating interventions or processes that teach palliative care professionals new skills, such as conflict management, interpersonal relationship development, or mindfulness, they may incorporate this knowledge into all aspects of their lives. Beyond employing newly learned mindfulness (see Box 7.17 for mindfulness suggestions related to the delivery of palliative care) in the workplace, PCT members will also benefit by using these skills in their personal life. Bottom line: A skills-based approach may help to increase provider self-care and well-being in and out of the workplace.

BOX 7.17

INTEGRATING MINDFUL COMMUNICATION IN PALLIATIVE CARE

Mindfulness describes a state where individuals stay focused and attuned to the present moment. While this sounds easy enough, consider how often you mentally return to your to-do list, consider what to make for dinner, and revisit that disagreement you had with your partner the night before. Following are some mindful communication practices shared by palliative care physicians.

Key Practice: Consider your audience(s).

In the day in and day out practice of palliative care, it can be easy to forget the magnitude of your role. As one palliative care clinician acknowledged: "When I first started out, I thought I knew best. I'd walk up to a patient, I'd already reviewed their chart, and I thought I knew them. I went on like this until my mentor told me, 'It's not about you. It's about them. You never even considered how they feel. … Just be there with them.' It was humbling and at the time, humiliating and infuriating, but the single most important piece of advice I've ever received. It's also the first lesson I teach new residents" (Omilion-Hodges & Swords, 2016, pp. 331).

Key Practice: Ask questions. Listen. Repeat.

Bill, a physician and medical director of a palliative care unit, stresses the importance of authenticity in patient–provider relationships. In fact, he refers to authenticity as a "relational slingshot" because it leads to "mutual and trusting relationships" and rapport development with patients (p. 331). Relatedly, Linda, a palliative care physician, suggests that she "scrutinizes" her early encounters with new patients so that she can tailor her communication, because they "walk this path together." The point of this key practice is to be fully present in patient encounters and not be perceived as just going through the motions of standard procedures. In Bill's advice to new residents: "be authentic even if they [new residents] are authentically awkward or shy or quiet. Whatever it is, as long as it is them and they are fully present in the conversation" (p. 331).

Key Practice: Discard scripts.

"We encourage our physicians to run to conflict, not away from it. We even provide bad death stories so they can learn. But we never provide a script. Even if it's not perfect, people can tell they're trying," stated Jim a palliative care physician (pp. 331–332). While scripts may be a helpful educational tool to provide students and residents with the scaffolding for challenging conversations, palliative care professionals should never be perceived as delivering a memorized cookie-cutter speech.

Key Practice: Recognize your role.

The final key mindful communication practice combines the three previous strategies. Lynn, a medical director of a palliative care unit, helped to illuminate this idea by reminding PCT members: "Whether you like it or not, or whether you're conscious of it or not, you're part of their [the patient and their family's] story" (p. 332). Remaining mindful and present with each patient can help you remember that while it is a normal Tuesday for you, it is likely a life-changing day for your patients and their family members. Lynn suggested that as PCT members complete their role-related duties that they remember that they're "a main character" in their patients' stories (p. 332).

SOURCE: American Hospital Association. (2019). *Circle of life criteria*. Retrieved from http://www.aha .org/about/awards/col/criteria.shtml; Omilion-Hodges, L. M., & Swords, N. M. (2016). Communication that heals: Mindful communication practices from palliative care leaders. *Health Communication, 31*(3), 328–335. doi:10.1080/10410236.2014.953739

PEARLS FROM THE FIELD: PROVIDER AND TEAM TAKEAWAYS

Palliative care professionals who practice self-care report a higher quality of life than peers who do not make self-care a priority. In addition to being more content in life, those who practice self-care are taking proactive measures to guard against the harmful effects of compassion fatigue and burnout.

Takeaway 1: Palliative care is challenging, emotionally intensive work.

Palliative care requires PCT members to comfort, support, and care for those with terminal, serious, and chronic illnesses day in and day out. In addition to

(continued next page)

these job-related charges, palliative care professionals are called to be adept communicators and relationship builders, often forging deep and meaningful connections with their patients and their patients' families. These meaningful relationships with patients can be both a sustaining and a draining part of being a palliative provider. Consistently witnessing the suffering and grief of others is challenging, and it becomes even more challenging when PCT members are expected to act in normative ways—remaining professional—when they are hurting or dealing with loss. Considering that getting to know, caring for, and going through the highs and lows of illness with patients is the cycle of palliative care, it is essential that PCT members develop healthy coping mechanisms, such as routine self-care measures, to bolster compassion satisfaction and to guard against burnout and compassion fatigue.

Takeaway 2: Self-care is an individual and team priority.

Palliative care professionals are responsible for integrating self-care into their personal and professional lives. As noted earlier, self-care has been identified as an essential practice for provider well-being by the Hospice and Palliative Medicine subspecialty. Through self-reflection, consideration of the dimensions of self-care, and creating a personalized self-care plan, PCT members can help to shield themselves from some of the challenges associated with the profession. However, this should not fall solely on individual PCT members (A self-care plan template is available at www.springerpub.com/palliativecareteam and at connect.springerpub.com/content/book/978-0-5806-2/ch07.). Team leaders should also consider meaningful ways of integrating self-care into the workplace and by cultivating a supportive team environment. Whether it is by shielding members from challenging work conditions, advocating for adequate resources, holding regular trainings related to personal (i.e., communication training) and professional (i.e., team stress reduction) development, or assigning work buddies or mentors, team leaders are in an influential position to help to create a workplace that allows members to focus on care delivery and not common organizational headaches.

References

American Hospital Association. (2019). *Circle of life criteria*. Retrieved from http://www.aha.org/about/awards/col/criteria.shtml

Anthony, M. K., & Vidal, K. (2010). Mindful communication: A novel approach to improving delegation and increasing patient safety. *OJIN: The Online Journal of Issues in Nursing, 15*(2). doi:10.3912/OJIN.Vol15No2Man02

Ayala, E. E., Omorodion, A. M., Nmecha, D., Winseman, J. S., & Mason, H. R. C. (2017). What do medical students do for self-care? A student-centered approach to well-being. *Teaching and Learning in Medicine: An International Journal, 29*(3), 237–246. doi:10.10 80/10401334.2016.1271334

Ayala, E. E., Winseman, J. S., Johnsen, R. D., & Mason, H. R. C. (2018). U.S. medical students who engage in self-care report less stress and higher quality of life. *BMC Medical Education, 18*(1), 189. doi:10.1186/s12909-018-1296-x

Back, A. L., Rushton, C. H., Kaszniak, A. W., & Halifax, J. S. (2015). "Why are we doing this?": Clinician helplessness in the face of suffering. *Journal of Palliative Medicine, 18*(1), 26–30. doi:10.1089/jpm.2014.0115

Back, A. L., Steinhauser, K. E., Kamal, A. H., & Jackson, V. A. (2016). Building resilience for palliative care clinicians: An approach to burnout prevention based on individual skills and workplace factors. *Journal of Pain and Symptom Management, 52*, 284–291. doi:10.1016/j.jpainsymman.2016.02.002

Balch, C. M., & Copeland, E. (2007). Stress and burnout among surgical oncologists: A call for personal wellness and a supportive workplace environment. *Annals of Surgical Oncology, 14*(11), 3029–3032. doi:10.1245/s10434-007-9588-0

Beckman, H. B., Wendland, M., Mooney, C., Krasner, M. S., Quill, T. E., Suchman, A. L., & Epstein, R. M. (2012). The impact of a program in mindful communication on primary care physicians. *Academic Medicine, 87*, 815–819. doi:10.1097/ACM.0b013e318253d3b2

Berman, R., Campbell, M., Makin, W., & Todd, C. (2007). Occupational stress in palliative medicine, medical oncology and clinical oncology specialist registrars. *Clinical Medicine, 7*, 235–242. doi:10.7861/clinmedicine.7-3-235

Boyle, D. A. (2011). Countering compassion fatigue : A requisite nursing agenda. *The Online Journal of Issues in Nursing, 16*(1), 1–13. doi:10.3912/OJIN.Vol16No01Man02

Brotheridge, C. M., & Grandey, A. A. (2002). Emotional labor and burnout: Comparing two perspectives of "people work". *Journal of Vocational Behavior, 60*, 17–39. doi:10.1006/jvbe.2001.1815

Burgoon, J. K., Berger, C. R., & Waldron, V. R. (2000). Mindfulness and interpersonal communication. *Journal of Social Issues, 56*(1), 105–127. doi:10.1111/0022-4537.00154

Carton, E. R., & Hupcey, J. E. (2014). The forgotten mourners: Addressing health care provider grief—A systematic review. *Journal of Hospice & Palliative Nursing, 16*(5), 291–303.

Cavallo, J. (2014). *Survey finds high rates of burnout among palliative care physicians, with over 50% predicted to leave the field in 10 years.* Retrieved from https://www.ascopost .com/News/19602

Cialdini, R. B. (2009). *Influence: Science and practice* (Vol. 4). Boston: Pearson Education.

Considine, J., & Miller, K. (2010). The dialectics of care: Communicative choices at the end of life. *Health Communication, 25*, 165–174. doi:10.1080/10410230903544951

Cross, L. A. (2019). Compassion fatigue in palliative care nursing: A concept analysis. *Journal of Hospice and Palliative Nursing, 21*(1), 21–28. doi:10.1097/NJH.0000000000000477

Dahlin, C., Coyne, P., Goldberg, J., & Vaughan, L. (2019). Palliative care leadership. *Journal of Palliative Care, 34*, 21–28. doi:10.1177/0825859718791427

Dahlin, C., Mastrojohn, J., & Rotella, J. (2018, March). Critical conversations: Challenges to clinician well-being and resilience in hospice and palliative care. In I. C. Fineberg (Moderator), *Town hall with AAHPM, HPNA, and NHPCO.* Symposium conducted at the Annual Assembly of Hospice and Palliative Care, Boston, MA.

Davidson, J. E., Graham, P., Montross-Tomas, L., Norcross, W., & Zerbi, G. (2017). Code lavender: Cultivating intentional acts of kindness in response to stressful work situations. *Explore, 13*(3), 181–185. doi:10.1016./j.explore.2017.02.005

Disch, J. (2018). Rethinking mentoring. *Critical Care Medicine, 46*(3), 437–441. doi:10.1097/CCM.0000000000002914

Funk, L. M., Peters, S., & Roger, K. S. (2017). The emotional labor of personal grief in palliative care: Balancing caring and professional identities. *Qualitative Health Research, 72*(14), 2211–2221. doi:10.1177/1049732317729139

Harrison, R. L., & Westwood, M. J. (2009). Preventing vicarious traumatization of mental health therapists: Identifying protective practices. *Psychotherapy: Theory, Research, Practice, Training, 46*(2), 203–219. doi:10.1037/a0016081

Joinson, C. (1992). Coping with compassion fatigue. *Nursing, 22*(4), 116–118.

Kabat-Zinn, J. (2006). Mindfulness-based interventions in context: Past, present, and future. *Clinical Psychology: Science and Practice, 10*(2), 144–156. doi:10.1093/clipsy.bpg016

Kamal, A. H., Bull, J. H., Wolf, M. S., Swetz, K. M., Shanafelt, T. D., Ast, K., … Abernathy, A. P. (2016). Prevalence and predictors of burnout among hospice and palliate care clinicians in the U.S. *Journal of Pain and Symptom Management, 51*(4), 690–696. doi:10.1016/j.jpainsymman.2015.10.020

Kearney, M. K., Weininger, R. B., Vachon, M. L., Harrison, R. L., & Mount, B. M. (2009). Self-care of physicians caring for patients at the end of life: "Being connected… a key to my survival." *The Journal of the American Medical Association, 301*(11), 1155–1164. doi:10.1001/jama.2009.352

Martins Pereira, S., Fonseca, A. M., & Sofia Carvalho, A. (2011). Burnout in palliative care: A systematic review. *Nursing Ethics, 18*(3), 317–326. doi:10.1177/0969733011398092

Mehta, D. H., Perez, G. K., Traeger, L., Park, E. R., Goldman, R. E., Haime, V., … Jackson, V. A. (2016). Building resiliency in a palliative care team: A pilot study. *Journal of Pain and Symptom Management, 51*, 604–608. doi:10.1016/j.jpainsymman.2015.10.013

Melvin, C. S. (2015). Historical review in understanding burnout, professional compassion fatigue, and secondary traumatic stress disorder from a hospice and palliative nursing perspective. *Journal of Hospice & Palliative Nursing, 17*, 66–72. doi:10.1097/NJH.0000000000000126

Miller, K. I. (2007). Compassionate communication in the workplace: Exploring processes of noticing, connecting, and responding. *Journal of Applied Communication Research, 35*, 223–245. doi:10.1080/ 00909880701434208

Mooney, C., Fetter, K., Gross, B. W., Rinehart, C., Lynch, C., & Rogers, F. B. (2017). A preliminary analysis of compassion satisfaction and compassion fatigue with considerations for nursing unit specialization and demographic factors. *Journal of Trauma Nursing, 24*(3), 158–163. doi:10.1097/JTN.0000000000000284

Nancarrow, S. A., Booth, A., Ariss, S., Smith, T., Enderby, P., & Roots, A. (2013). Ten principles of good interdisciplinary team work. *Human Resources for Health, 11*, 11–19. doi:10.1186/1478-4491-11-19

National Sleep Foundation. (2015, February 2). *National sleep foundation recommends new sleep times* [Press release]. Retrieved from https://www.sleepfoundation.org/press-release/national-sleep-foundation-recommends-new-sleep-times

O'Connor, N. (2018, January 19). *Consults, consults, and more consults: Strategies for managing inpatient demand in excess of staffing* [web log comment]. Retrieved from https://www.capc.org/blog/palliative-pulse-palliative-pulse-january-2018-strategies-managing-inpatient-demand/

Omilion-Hodges, L. M., & Ackerman, C. D. (2018). From the technical know-how to the free flow of ideas: Exploring the effects of leader, peer, and team communication on employee creativity. *Communication Quarterly, 66*(1), 38–57. doi:10.1080/01463373 .2017.1325385

Omilion-Hodges, L. M., & Swords, N. M. (2016). Communication that heals: Mindful communication practices from palliative care leaders. *Health Communication, 31*(3), 328–335. doi:10.1080/10410236.2014.953739

Palliative Dork [@PCDorkClub]. Tweets: 5/29/19, 5/14/19, 4/5/19. Retrieved from https://twitter.com/PCDorkClub

Sanchez-Reilly, S., Morrison, L. J., Carey, E., Bernacki, R., O'Neill, L., Kapo, J., ... deLima Thomas, J. (2013). Caring for oneself to care for others: Physicians and their self-care. *The Journal of Supportive Oncology, 11*(2), 75–81. Retrieved from https://www.ncbi.nlm.nih.gov/pmc/articles/PMC3974630/

Sans, N., Galiana, L., Oliver, A., Pascual, A., Sinclair, S., & Benito, E. (2015). Palliative care professionals' inner life: Exploring the relationships among awareness, self-care, and compassion satisfaction and fatigue, burnout, and coping with death. *Journal of Pain and Symptom Management, 50*, 200–207. doi:10.1016/j.jpainsymman.2015.02.013

Shanafelt, T. D., West, C. P., Sloan, J. A., Novotny, P. J., Poland, G. A., Menaker, R., ... Drybye, L. N. (2009). Career fit and burnout among academic faculty. *Archives of Internal Medicine 169*(10), 990–995. doi:10.1001/archinternmed.2009.70

Shanafelt, T. D., West, C. P., Zhao, X., Novotny, P., Kolars, J., Habermann, T., & Sloan, J. (2005). Relationship between increased personal well-being and enhanced empathy among. *Journal of General Internal Medicine, 20*(7), 559–564. doi:10.1007/s11606-005-0102-8

Sims, S., Hewitt, G., & Harris, R. (2015). Evidence of collaboration, pooling of resources, learning and role blurring in interprofessional healthcare teams: A realist synthesis. *Journal of Interprofessional Care, 29*(1), 20–25. doi:10.3109/13561820.2014.939745

Sorenson, C., Bolick, B., Wright, K., & Hamilton, R. (2016). Understanding compassion fatigue in healthcare providers: A review of current literature. *Journal of Nursing Scholarship, 48*(5), 456–465. doi:10.1111/jnu.12229

Spilman, J. (2010, November 1). *Cumulative grief in healthcare professionals* [web log comment]. Retrieved from https://caregiverwellness.blogspot.com/2010/11/cumulative-grief-in-healthcare.html

Swetz, K. M., Harrington, S. E., Matsuyama, R. K., Shanafelt, T. D., & Lyckholm, L. J. (2009). Strategies for avoiding burnout in hospice and palliative medicine: Peer advice for physicians on achieving longevity and fulfillment. *Journal of Palliative Medicine, 12*(9), 773–777. doi:10.1089/jpm.2009.0050

Vedel, I., Ghadi, V., Lapointe, L., Routelous, C., Aegerter, P., & Guirimand, F. (2014). Patients', family caregivers', and professionals' perspectives on quality of palliative care: A qualitative study. *Palliative Medicine, 28*(9), 1128–1138. doi:10.1177/0269216314532154.

West, C. P., Huschka, M. M., Novotny, P. J., Sloan, J. A., Kolars, J. C., Habermann, T. M., & Shanafelt, T. D. (2006). Association of perceived medical errors with resident distress and empathy: A prospective longitudinal study. *The Journal of the American Medical Association, 296*(9), 1071–1078. doi:10.1001/jama.296.9.1071

INDEX

ACHPN. *See* Advanced Certified Hospice and Palliative Nurse
active listening, 15–16, 19, 185, 204
administrative coordination meetings, 140, 151
administrative leaders, 46–47, 100, 102, 106
Advanced Certified Hospice and Palliative Care Nurse (ACHPN), 39
advanced practice providers (APPs), 38–40
advanced practice registered nurse (APRNs), 37, 38–40, 77, 78, 79, 80, 89
advocacy, leadership in, 102
aging population, and demand for palliative care, 5–6
American Board of Medical Specialties, 37
American Nurses Association (ANA), 40
American Nurses Credentialing Center (ANCC), 115
American Society of Clinical Oncology (ASCO), 4
American Society of Health-System Pharmacists (ASHP), Guidelines on the Pharmacist's Role in Palliative and Hospice Care, 45
ANA. *See* American Nurses Association
ANCC. *See* American Nurses Credentialing Center
Annual Assembly of Hospice and Palliative Care, 210
APPs. *See* advanced practice providers
APRNs. *See* advanced practice registered nurse
ASCO. *See* American Society of Clinical Oncology
ASHP. *See* American Society of Health-System Pharmacists, Guidelines on the Pharmacist's Role in Palliative and Hospice Care

Association of Professional Chaplains Code of Ethics, 43
authenticity, in patient–provider relationship, 223–224

baby boomers, 5
BCCs. *See* board-certified chaplains
billing structures, 53, 115, 116
biomedical model of medicine, 53, 161, 164, 173, 175, 182
biopsychosocial model of medicine, 161, 164, 174–175, 175, 182, 184
board-certified chaplains (BCCs), 43
body language, and active listening, 16
boundaries, 70, 72
 and decision-making, 164
 occupational, 162, 164
 respecting, 48
 setting, 216–217
breathing exercise, 212, 214
burnout, 22, 197–198, 199, 200, 201.
  See also self-care
 causes of, 202
 and communication, 19
 vs. compassion fatigue, 202–203
 outcomes of, 203
 and staffing, 11, 85
 and surface acting, 195–196
 timing of, 202
 for underresourced palliative care staff, 201, 203–204
 and workplace environment, 217, 218

CAPC. *See* Center to Advance Palliative Care
CDC. *See* Centers for Disease Control and Prevention
Center to Advance Palliative Care (CAPC), 2, 24, 51, 127, 183
 impact calculator, 12

Centers for Disease Control and
    Prevention (CDC), 5
certification, palliative care, 37
certified nurse midwife (CNM), 39
certified registered nurse anesthetist
    (CRNA), 39
chaplains, 37, 43–44, 102, 177, 206, 214
    engagement with patients, 52
    occupational culture of, 165
    role clarity, 47, 49, 51–52
clinical leaders, 46–47, 55, 100, 101, 103, 106
clinical nurse practitioner (CNP), 39
clinical nurse specialist (CNS), 39
Clinical Pastoral Education (CPE), 43
*Clinical Practice Guidelines for Quality
    Palliative Care*, 4th edition, 3, 35
CNM. *See* certified nurse midwife
CNP. *See* clinical nurse practitioner
CNS. *See* clinical nurse specialist
Code Lavender, 210
cognitive dissonance, 126
cognitive mapping, 69
cohesive communication, 83–84
COMFORT model, 19
communication, 24, 27, 69, 72, 94, 130, 133
    alternative ways, 78
    face-to-face, 149–152, 157
    focus on, 3
    foundational role of, 14–15, 185, 187
        in healthcare environment, 15–21
    gaps, and peer relationships, 180, 181
    hubs, 85–86
    intentional, 12–14, 86–87, 112,
        117–123, 178, 185
    interdisciplinary, 166–167, 187
    and length of stay, 10–11
    and power differentials, 53–54
    processing, 82–83
    serpentine conversations, 75–78
community challenges of palliative care
    teams, 182–185
compassion fatigue, 199–200, 201, 209.
        See also self-care
    vs. burnout, 202–203
    causes of, 202
    circumstances, 199–200
    contributors to, 200

lasting effects of, 201
moral distress, 205–210
outcomes of, 200, 202
progressive nature of, 201
secondary traumatic stress, 205
timing of, 202
workflow strategies for overworked
    programs, 208–209
compassion satisfaction, 198–199, 209
conflict(s), 48, 94
    in decision-making, 70
    destructive, 27, 73, 93
    group, 139
    interpersonal, dealing with, 79
    management, 73, 220
    productive, 73, 92, 93, 94, 139
consensus building, 81, 91–94, 139
constructive conflict, 73
constructive marginalization, 90–91
Coordinated Management of Meaning
    Model, 75–78
CPE. *See* Clinical Pastoral Education
CRNA. *See* certified registered nurse
    anesthetists
cumulative grief, 205

data management, 128–129
death
    contradictory views of, 181–182
    good, 3, 168, 178, 182, 188, 205
    of patients, acknowledging, 206
    quality of, 7
debate, 74
decision-making, 25, 184
    consensus in, 92, 139
    devil's advocate, 137
    effect of group harmony, productive/
        destructive conflict on, 93
    family, 155–156
    and groupthink, 138
    obstruction, 139
    and occupational boundaries, 164
    and physicians, 53
    and storytelling, 168
    and transparent communication,
        120–121

deep acting, 195, 197, 198
demand for palliative care, 4–5, 187
    aging population, 5–6
    growth of PCTs, 7–8
    and improved clinical outcomes, 6–7
destructive conflict, 27, 73
    effect on team decision-making, 93
devil's advocate, in meetings, 137
dialogue, 74
discharge planning, 41–42
discussion, 74
disruptors, 139
dissent, 90–91
    communication of, 107
    and decision-making, 73, 92, 121
    handling, in team meetings, 138–139
    vs. obstruction, 121, 139
domains of care, 34, 35

education, palliative care, 23–26, 161
    Clinical Pastoral Education, 43
    leadership in, 102
ego, 72, 76, 109
electronic medical record (EMR), 150
email, 107
emotional labor, 14, 19, 22, 191. See also
        self-care
    employee-focused, 195–198
    and humor, 196–197
    -intensive positions, 192–193
    job-focused, 194–195
    meaningful work, 193, 198, 201
    social media as support, 196
empathy, 16, 216–217, 217
employee-focused emotional labor,
        195–198
EMR. See electronic medical record
encrypted messaging, 150
environment, workplace, 217–219
equivocality of palliative care, 21, 25, 70
explanatory uncertainty, 68
exquisite empathy, 216–217

face-to-face communication, 149–152, 157
fake consensus, 91–92

Family Meeting Assessment Tool (FMAT),
        154
family meetings, 152–156
fiscal savings for hospitals, 8, 9–12
FMAT. See Family Meeting Assessment
        Tool
formal leaders, 46, 55, 100, 101, 103, 106,
        107, 129
formal team meetings, 141, 143–144,
        151–152
forming stage, team formation, 67, 69–72
funding for team and provider
        development, 183

goals
    coordination of, 135–136
    goal-concordant care, 133, 136, 140,
        144–145
    team-based, 87–88
Gold Standards Framework, 25
grief, 192, 193, 194
    cumulative, 205
ground rules, meeting, 136
group conflicts, 139
group harmony, effect on team decision-
        making, 93
group identity, 63, 75, 114
groupthink, 92, 138

happy hour, 89, 142
Health Professionals Core
        Communication Curriculum
        (HPCCC), 13
helplessness, feeling of, 205–210
hidden profiles, and decision-making, 92
high-performing palliative care teams, 9,
        25, 156
high-reliability organizations, 22
holiday party, 142
Hospice and Palliative Medicine
        fellowship program, 37
HPCCC. See Health Professionals Core
        Communication Curriculum
humor, expression/uses of, 89, 126,
        196–197

I can't phrase, using, 121, 122
identity politics, 114–115, 117
immediacy behaviors, 110–111
imposter syndrome, 126
informal leaders, 46, 100–101, 106, 129
informal team meetings, 141–142,
    148–149, 151–152
information sharing, 79, 92
ingroups, 63
    communication, 69, 71
    double ingroup members, 80
    humor, 89
    identification of, 70
    partial ingroup members, 80
Institute of Medicine (IOM), 23
    Dying in America report, 8, 23
    Future of Nursing report, 41
integrative medicine, 11
intentional communication, 12–14, 86–87,
    112, 117–123, 178, 185
intentional communities, 86–87, 88
    consensus building, 91–94
    constructive marginalization, 90–91
    shared/negotiated value system, 88–90
    team-based goals, achievement of,
        87–88
intentional language usage, 15, 16, 185
interdisciplinary communication,
    166–167, 187
interdisciplinary teams, 2, 8, 24, 33, 35, 65,
    70, 82, 91, 135, 161
    and communication, 17, 24
    fiscal savings for hospitals, 8, 9–12
    formation. *See* team formation/
        maintenance
    meetings. *See* team meetings
    minimally performing *vs.* high-
        performing PCTs, 9
    return on investment, 11
    role clarity. *See* role clarity, in palliative
        care teams
interfaith chaplains, 43
interpersonal relationship, 72, 219
interpretive models, 172, 174
    biomedical model of medicine, 53, 161,
        164, 173, 175, 182

biopsychosocial model of medicine,
    161, 164, 174–175, 175, 182, 184
IOM. *See* Institute of Medicine

jargon, 163
job-focused emotional labor, 194–195

knowledge gaps, and peer relationships,
    179–180, 181

language. *See* intentional language usage
leader–member relationship, 120
    impact on peer relationships, 113
    perception questions about, 107
    role making, 108
    role routinization, 108
    role taking, 108
leadership, definitions of, 101
leadership, palliative care team, 46–47, 99–
    100, 101–102, 129–130, 170–171
    characteristics, 100
    and conflict management, 73
    importance of team leaders, 106–117
    modeling intentional, relational
        communication, 117–123
    new team members, selection/
        orientation of, 123, 124–126
    perceptions, managing
        larger organization, 114–117
        relationships/resources, 113
    problem-solving, 103, 104–106
    relationships, managing, 106–107
    resources, managing, 107–112
    team changes, leading through, 124–126
    team member who is not good fit,
        handling, 126–127
    team outcomes, management of,
        127–129
location of palliative care units, 183, 184
logistics, and texting, 150
lunch
    skipping, consequences of, 216
    team lunch, 141, 148–149, 183

Magnet® status, 115
marketing, 183, 222
meaning-centered approach to
    communication, 16–17, 18–19, 185
meaningful work, 193, 198, 201
medical system, flaws in, 22–23, 165
meetings. *See also* team meetings
  assumptions about, 142
  types of, 141–142
mentorship/mentoring, 5, 40, 41, 117, 219
mindful communication, 91, 140, 221,
    223–224
  in meetings, 142–143, 146
mindfulness, 214, 215, 220–221, 223
minimally performing palliative care
    teams, 9
mission moments, 222
mobile phones/electronic devices, 149
  and immediacy, 110, 111–112
  texting, 111–112, 149, 150–151
moral distress, 205–210
morning table rounds. *See* patient
    coordination meetings
multidisciplinary teams, 64, 135. *See also*
    interdisciplinary teams

name calling, 179, 187
National Comprehensive Cancer Network
    (NCCN), 55
National Consensus Project (NCP), 2, 3,
    35
NCCN. *See* National Comprehensive
    Cancer Network
NCP. *See* National Consensus Project
negative resources, 107, 109–110, 113
nonverbal immediacy behaviors, 110–111
norming stage, team formation, 68, 81
  bonded believers and
      interdependent
      interdisciplinarians, 82–83
  cohesive communication, 83–84
  communication point people, 85–86
  processing communication, 82–83
  unexpected absence, dealing with, 85
  value, communicating, 84–85

obstruction, distinguishing dissent from,
    121, 139
occupational culture, 161–163, 175–178, 187
  contradictory views of death, 181–182
  difficult organizational environments,
      surviving, 185
  impact on interdisciplinary
      collaboration, 163–166
  interdisciplinary communication,
      166–167
  interdisciplinary peer relationships,
      challenges in, 178–181
  living–dying tension, 175–176
  organizational and community
      challenges, 182–185
  practicing–advocating tension, 176,
      177–178
  storytelling, 167–172
  teaching colleagues about palliative
      care, 177
  tensions between palliative care
      providers and other medical
      providers, 172–175
occupational identity, 162–163, 169, 193
occupational socialization, 163–164, 165,
    178, 187
oncology
  clinicians, interdisciplinary experience
      of, 24
  reduction in cost of care, 10
  tumor boards, 174
organizational culture, 123, 124, 184, 185
organization(s), 22, 125
  accrediting, 115
  challenges, 182–185, 187–188
  complex, problem-solving in, 25
  difficult environments, surviving in, 185
  high-reliability, 22
  perceptions, managing, 114–117
  politics, 114
  sensemaking process in, 22, 70
  transparency in, 120
orientation of new team members, 123,
    124–126
other-oriented approach to
    communication, 16, 185

outcomes measurement, 127–129
outgroups, 63
    communication, 69, 71, 86
    and discrimination, 90
    double outgroup members, 80
    identification of, 70
    negative interaction with, 73
    partial outgroup members, 80
    serpentine conversations, 75, 76
outreach, leadership in, 102

PAHPM. *See* Physician Assistants in
        Hospice and Palliative Medicine
palliative care, 1, 2, 27
    ambiguity in system and teams, 21–23
    different lenses of, 36
    for family members of healthcare
        providers, 178
    focus on team and communication in, 3
    improved clinical outcomes with, 6
    increasing demand for, 4–8
    negative experience, 1–2, 33, 61, 99,
        133, 162, 191–192
    new hires, 183
    positive experience, 2, 33, 35, 61–62,
        100, 134, 162, 192
    practice, misunderstandings about, 154
    primary, 4
    resource allocation for, 7
    specialty, 4
    teaching colleagues about, 177
    training and education, 23–26
    understanding of, 23
palliative care specialists, 35, 37
    advanced practice providers, 38–40
    chaplains, 43–44
    and other medical providers, tensions
        between, 172–175
    pharmacists, 44–45
    physicians, 37–38
    registered nurses, 40–41
    social workers, 41–42
palliative care teams (PCTs), 2, 3, 5, 21,
        26–27, 56
    average salaries of members, 54
    conceptualization of, 24

formation/maintenance. *See* team
        formation/maintenance
    growth of, 7–8
    health, threats to, 102–103
    high-performing, 9, 25
    interaction with multidisciplinary
        hospital departments, 62–63
    members, well-being of. *See* self-care;
        team care
    minimally performing, 9
    negotiations of, 183–184
    organizational preparation for, 69
    physical location of, 183, 184
    power differentials within, 52–55, 56–57
    well-being/collective functioning,
        factors that enhance, 218
parallel storytelling, 83–84, 93–94
paraphrasing, and active listening, 16
PAs. *See* physician assistants
patient-centered care, 6, 17, 19, 62, 65,
        103, 181
patient coordination meetings, 38, 103,
        140, 141, 144–148
    example, 146–148
    and family members, 152–153
    functions of, 146
    identification of member strengths, 148
    roles for members, 147, 148
    tasks, 147, 148
    team communication considerations,
        145–146
PCTs. *See* palliative care teams
pediatric palliative care teams (PPCTs), 26
peer relationships, 178, 219
    impact of leader–member relationship
        on, 113
    interdisciplinary, challenges in, 178–179
        communication gaps, 180, 181
        knowledge gaps, 179–180, 181
        value gaps, 180, 181
performing stage, team formation, 68,
        86–87, 124
personal tendencies/preferences, reflection
        of leaders on, 107, 120
personal worth, and self-care, 213
personality conflicts, 48
pharmacists, 37, 44–45, 51, 101

physical health, and self-care, 213
physical proximity of team members, 136, 151
physician assistants (PAs), 38–40
Physician Assistants in Hospice and Palliative Medicine (PAHPM), 38
physicians, 37–38, 102
    as experts, positioning, 164–165
    occupational culture of, 165
    occupational socialization of, 163–164
    and power differentials, 52–55, 56–57, 72
    and shared leadership, 54–55, 56
policy, leadership in, 102
POLST. See Practitioner Orders for Life Sustaining Treatment
positive resources, 107, 109, 113
power
    differentials within palliative care teams, 52–55, 56–57
        and forming stage, 72
        and norming stage, 89
        and identity politics, 114, 115
PPCTs. See pediatric palliative care teams
Practitioner Orders for Life Sustaining Treatment (POLST), 40
predictive uncertainty, 68
primary palliative care, 4
primary traumatic stress, 205
problem-solving, 88
    in complex organizations, 25
    and physical proximity of team members, 151
    requisite variety, 25, 70, 151
    and shared leadership, 103, 104–106
    and team-based care, 19–21, 23
    and team meetings, 134–135
productive conflicts, 73, 94, 139
    effect on team decision-making, 92, 93
public relations, 183

QODD. See Quality of Death and Dying Scale
QOL. See quality of life
Quality of Death and Dying Scale (QODD), 7
quality of life (QOL), 4, 6, 178, 210

of palliative care providers, 200, 211–212, 224

rank order system, 53, 164–165
reference group, 163
referrals to palliative care, 23, 25–26, 103, 154
registered nurses (RNs), 37, 40–41, 49, 126–127, 166
relational meaning of conversations, and texting, 150
relationship(s)
    agendas, and team meetings, 138
    and communication of leaders, 117, 118–120
    conflict, 139
    interdisciplinary peer relationships, challenges in, 178–181
    interpersonal, 72, 219
    leader–member relationship, 120
        development, 108
        impact on peer relationships, 113
        perception questions about, 107
    management by leaders, 106–107
    perceptions, managing, 113
    personal tendencies/preferences, reflection on, 107, 120
    and physical proximity of team members, 136, 151
    social, 163
RENEW model, 19, 207–208
reporting structure, 115, 116
requisite variety, 25, 70, 151
research, leadership in, 102, 103
resources
    allocation
        for palliative care, 7, 184
        and power differentials, 53
        and storytelling, 171
        tensions, 182
    burnout for underresourced palliative care staff, 201, 203–204
    management of, 107–112
    negative, 107, 109–110, 113
    perceptions, managing, 113
    positive, 107, 109, 113

respect, 48, 49, 51, 56, 89, 90
retreats, team, 140, 141, 144, 151, 183
retroactive sensemaking, 168
revenue generation, 53, 115
rituals, acknowledging death of patients
    through, 206
RNs. *See* registered nurses
road map for conducting family
    meetings, 154
role clarity, 47–51, 56
    challenges with borrowed team
        members, 51–52
    role blurring, 47, 118, 219
    role flexibility/flexing, 49, 51, 85,
        219
    team exercise for, 50
role model desired communication
    behaviors/practices, 121–123
rounds. *See* patient coordination
    meetings

Saunders, Cicely, 33, 35
secondary traumatic stress (STS), 205
self-care, 191, 199, 209, 210–211, 224–225.
    See also team care
    activities, 211–212, 214
    balancing individual needs in a team
        context, 213–215
    benefits of, 212–213
    consequences of skipping lunch and
        staying late, 216
    empathy and boundary setting, 216–217
    importance of, 213
    practice, integration into team
        environment, 222–224
sensemaking, 22, 70
    retroactive, 168
    and storytelling, 168
shared leadership, 46, 54–55, 56, 103,
    104–106
SIT. *See* social identity theory
skilled nursing facility (SNF), 20–21
skills-based approach to self-care, 223
smartphones. *See* mobile phones/
    electronic devices
SNF. *See* skilled nursing facility

social identity, 70, 162–163
social identity theory (SIT), 63, 70
social media, 196
social relationships, 163
social support
    and self-care, 215
    and work buddies, 219
social workers (SWs), 37, 41–42, 47,
    51, 53, 72, 77, 78, 102, 123,
    165, 197
socialization, occupational, 163–164, 165,
    178, 187
specialty palliative care, 4
SPIKES model, 154
spiritual assessment, 43, 47, 84
spiritual care, 43–44
spiritual history, 43
staffing, palliative care, 8, 136
    and burnout, 11, 85, 201, 203–204
Stamm, Beth Hudnall, 200
storming stage, team formation, 67, 68,
    73–81, 89, 90
storytelling, 167–168, 178, 188
    aspects to integrate into, 169
    by family members, 172
    parallel, 83–84, 93–94
    professional arc story, 170–171
    reasons for using, 168
    suggestions
        for new palliative care professionals,
        169–170
        for seasoned palliative care
        professionals, 170
        for students, 169
stress, 1, 85
    impact on well-being, 213
    management, and self-care, 212
    moments, talking through, 204
    primary traumatic stress, 205
    secondary traumatic stress, 205
structurational divergence theory,
    185, 186
STS. *See* secondary traumatic stress
suffering, 33
superordinate goals, 87–88, 135
surface acting, 195–196, 219
SWs. *See* social workers

table rounds. *See* patient coordination meetings
task agendas, and team meetings, 138
team-based care, 1, 3, 26, 63–64
  problem-solving, 19–21, 23
team bonding
  through processing experiences, 82
  and texting, 151
team care, 191, 210. *See also* self-care
  building, into effective teams, 217–224
  environmental factors, 218
  formalized team expectations, 219–220
  interpersonal relationship, 219
  mindfulness, 220–221
  mission moments, 222
  regular assessment, 222
  work load flexibility, 220
team culture, 103, 123, 124
team formation/maintenance, 65, 94, 156, 187
  adjourning stage, 68
  and disruptors, 139
  forming stage, 67, 69–72
    questions, 71
  intentional communities. *See* intentional communities
  nonpalliative care staff, alleviating distress of, 89
  norming stage, 68, 81–86
  outperforming, 68
  performing stage, 68, 86–87
  storming stage, 67, 68, 73–81
  and time commitment, 140
  Tuckman's stage model (1965), 65, 67, 124
team identity, 114–115, 117, 157
team meetings, 38, 53, 118, 133–134, 136, 141, 156–157
  advantages and disadvantages of, 136–138
  communication considerations, 145–146
  dissent, handling, 138–139
  family meetings, 152–156
  formal, 141, 143–144, 151–152
  informal, 141–142, 148–149, 151–152
  patient coordination meetings, 38, 103, 140, 141, 144–148
  and productivity/workloads, 157

task and relationship agendas, 138
time commitment, 140
virtual *vs.* face-to-face teamwork, 149–152
teamwork, 62–63, 185
  beyond multidisciplinary teams, 63–65
  virtual *vs.* face-to-face, 149–152
technology, 110, 111–112, 149–152, 156
texting, 111–112, 149, 150–151, 163
time commitment, 140
timekeeper, for meetings, 137, 147
total pain, 33
training, palliative care, 23–26, 161, 187
  and leadership, 103
  social workers, 41
transdisciplinary teams, 17, 24, 64, 65, 118, 135, 156. *See also* interdisciplinary teams
  and communication, 118
  direct communication in, 149
  evolution of healthcare to, 66
transparency in communication, 120–121
true consensus, 91
trust, 118, 209, 219
  and active listening, 16
  -based accountability model, 18
  and group membership, 79, 219
  and leader-member relationship, 108, 110, 112, 118
tumor boards, 174
turnover, palliative care team, 1, 26, 99, 111, 185
Twitter, 196

value(s), 81, 162, 163
  gaps, and peer relationships, 180, 181
  shared/negotiated value system, 88–90
vicarious trauma. *See* secondary traumatic stress (STS)
virtual communication, 149–152

word matching, 83
work buddies, 219
work performance, reflection on, 215
work styles, 72
work–life balance, 195, 209, 212

Printed in the United States
by Baker & Taylor Publisher Services